PELVIC FLOOR YOGA FOR WOMEN

PELVIC FLOOR YOGA for WOMEN

Simple Poses for Healing Your Body and Boosting Strength

CHRISTINA D'ARRIGO

ROCKRIDGE
PRESS

First Rockridge Press trade paperback edition 2022

Rockridge Press and the Rockridge Press logo are trademarks or registered trademarks of Callisto Media Inc. and/or its affiliates in the United States and other countries and may not be used without written permission.

For general information on our other products and services, please contact our Customer Care Department within the United States at (866) 744-2665, or outside the United States at (510) 253-0500.

Paperback ISBN: 978-1-63878-474-6 | eBook ISBN: 978-1-63878-654-2

Manufactured in the United States of America

Interior and Cover Designer: Lisa Forde
Art Producer: Melissa Malinowksy
Editor: Eun H. Jeong
Production Editor: Matthew Burnett
Production Manager: Riley Hoffman

Illustrations © 2022 Collaborate Agency; magemasher/123RF, p.7; all other illustrations used under license from Shutterstock.com

Author photograph courtesy of Allison Armfield

10 9 8 7 6 5 4 3 2 1 0

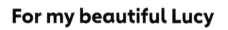
For my beautiful Lucy

Contents

Introduction

Welcome to your pelvic floor yoga journey! You've come to the right place to discover a renewed sense of healing, health, revitalization, and harmony in your body. I'm Christina, a yoga teacher based in New York City. I teach yoga, mainly online via my YouTube channel, *Yoga With Christina*, to thousands of people all over the world. I have 500 hours of yoga teacher training and bachelor's and master's degrees in dance choreography.

I learned a great deal about my pelvic floor after giving birth to my first child. During the postpartum period, I noticed that my pelvic floor was much weaker than it had been before pregnancy and labor. I learned that with time, patience, and dedication to a yoga practice, recovering the strength that I had lost in my pelvic floor was achievable.

You may have picked up this book because you are pregnant, or you just gave birth. Or perhaps you just want to strengthen your pelvic floor or feel more connected to it. You may also just be looking to improve your overall well-being. Whatever the reason or circumstance, this book aims to provide a comprehensive guide to support your journey of strengthening, revitalizing, and healing your pelvic floor. It does so by combining yoga and movement along with research-based practices for recovery from pregnancy and delivery.

If you feel uncomfortable with your pelvic floor muscles at the moment, know you do not have to feel this way forever. Just by picking up this book, you're on your way to improving your health and feeling more confident. Your body can heal and grow stronger with knowledge and dedication to the practice and yourself. You can take what you learn in this book to create a customized pelvic floor yoga practice that will help you achieve your goals. It will take time, discipline, and patience, but all that work is well worth the effort when you feel better overall!

Practicing yoga is a great way to add more positivity and light into your life, and just because you are doing it for a specific purpose does not mean that you won't reap the other benefits yoga has to offer, including flexibility, mental clarity, mindfulness, and an overall sense of well-being. I hope you enjoy this journey to a healthier and happier pelvic floor—and you!

How to Use This Book

This book is divided into two parts. Part 1 explains yoga and its benefits for your body and, specifically, the pelvic floor. You'll also learn about pelvic floor anatomy, what to look out for in terms of pelvic floor health, and how to practice pelvic floor yoga safely. Part 2 offers a collection of beginner-friendly pelvic floor–specific yoga poses and sequences that will help you strengthen and heal your pelvic floor muscles and support your body and overall health and well-being.

Each pose includes detailed instructions and illustrations on how to execute the pose, the benefits of the pose, tips for leveling up or adjusting for your comfort level, and any precautions you may need to take. In general, you should feel comfortable in these poses. If you do feel any sharp pain or discomfort in your joints, please skip that particular pose. For the sequences, you'll find guidance on how to move through the poses, as well as modification tips to adjust the sequence for your comfort.

The yoga poses in this book are drawn from hatha, vinyasa, restorative, and yin yoga techniques. Although each style of yoga is different, they all have great benefits for health, including building muscle and stamina and helping you relax.

Although this book is geared generally toward female yoga practitioners, it can be of service to anyone with a pelvic floor, regardless of sex and/or gender identification. If you are looking to improve and heal your pelvic floor muscles through a guided yoga practice, then this book is for you.

It's important to note that this book is not a replacement for medical advice from a professional health care practitioner. If you have undiagnosed pelvic floor pain or discomfort, always speak with a doctor for an accurate medical diagnosis and treatment plan.

Now, let's set off on your journey to a healthier and stronger pelvic floor!

PART I

ALL ABOUT PELVIC FLOOR YOGA

In this section, we'll explore what yoga is and what its benefits are, what the pelvic floor is and what it does for your body, what having a weak pelvic floor can mean, the benefits of having a strong pelvic floor, and the advantages of a regular pelvic floor yoga practice. We'll top things off with a quick exercise you can do on the go to strengthen your pelvic muscles. I will then offer some tips to prepare for a successful and comfortable pelvic floor yoga practice.

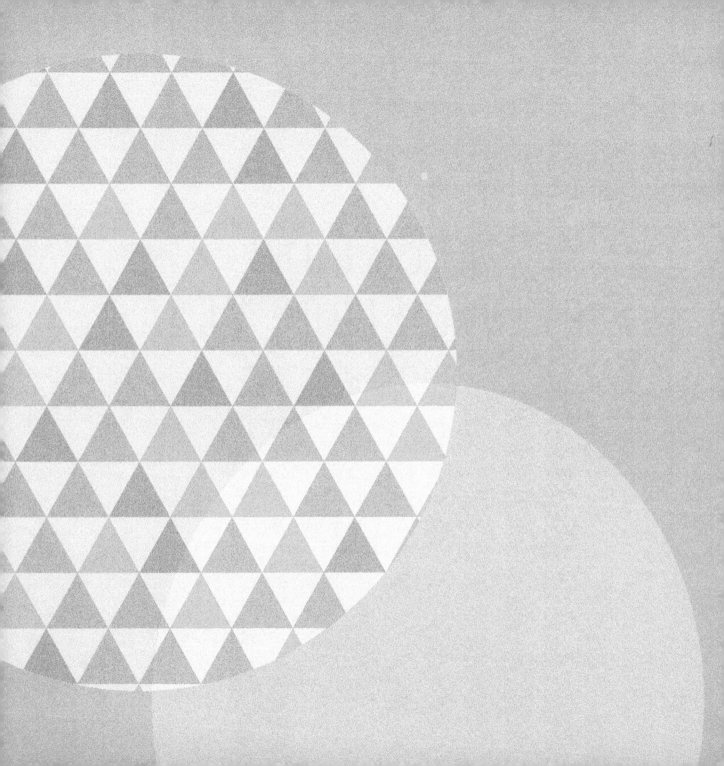

CHAPTER ONE

Getting Started with Pelvic Floor Yoga

This chapter is an introduction to yoga and the pelvic floor. It will explain how the two can work together to improve your overall health, well-being, vitality, strength, confidence, and self-esteem. We'll cover the basics of yoga and describe the muscles of the pelvic floor and their location. I will then share what it means to have a weak pelvic floor and how to go about strengthening the area through yoga.

Yoga for Body, Mind, and Spirit

Whether you are a beginner or a seasoned yogi, a regular yoga practice benefits your mind, body, and spirit in many ways.

There are no limits to the positive changes that you can gain. With a more restorative and restful type of yoga, you'll experience increased levels of relaxation from the activation of your body's resting state. A cardio-based yoga style promotes an increase in energy levels and vitality. Certain yoga poses improve balance and posture, whereas other yoga poses help build muscle strength or improve flexibility and joint mobility.

Yoga is much more than just physical exercise. Yoga means "union"—as such, it is meant to connect and unify the mind, body, and spirit. This also means that when practicing the yoga *asanas*—the physical postures of yoga—we enjoy mental benefits in addition to the physical benefits. With a regular yoga practice comes more mindfulness, mental clarity, and self-awareness. It's also common to feel more at peace and calm overall, even outside of your yoga practice.

Practicing yoga regularly is important for both short- and long-term benefits. Although it may be difficult to fit yoga into a busy schedule, a regular practice is necessary to see the positive change within yourself and achieve the results you want. But even just practicing one longer sequence once a week, or a shorter sequence every few days, will result in improvements in your health and well-being.

The Pelvic Floor

The pelvis, or pelvic bones, is formed by the two hip bones (left and right), the sacrum, and the coccyx (tailbone). The hip bone consists of the ilium, ischium, and pubis (pubic bone). The ischial tuberosity, sometimes referred to as the sit bones, is the lower part of your pelvis. The pelvic floor comprises a group of muscles deep at the bottom of the pelvis, running from the pubis at the front of the pelvis to the coccyx at the back.

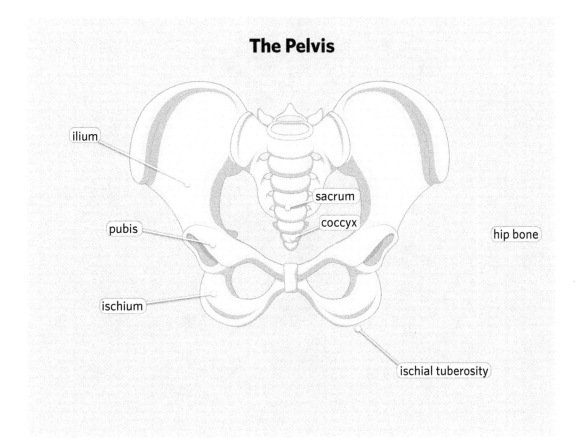

The Pelvis

ilium

sacrum

coccyx

pubis

hip bone

ischium

ischial tuberosity

In females, the pelvic floor muscles support all the organs of the pelvis: the anus, bladder, bowel, urethra, uterus, and vagina. These pelvic floor muscles hold these organs in place and assist in their proper functioning. Though several other important bones and structures make up the pelvis, these are often the main structures we deal with when discussing the pelvic floor.

The Organs of the Pelvis

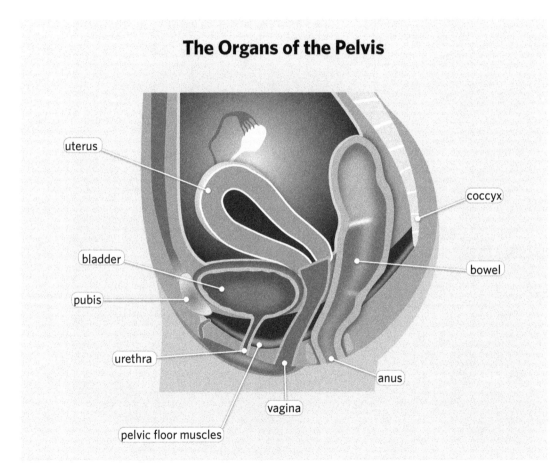

The outermost layer of pelvic floor muscles within the pelvic bones includes the bulbocavernosus, external anal sphincter, ischiocavernosus, and superficial transverse perineal muscle.

The middle layer is made up of the urethral sphincter, compressor urethrae, and deep transverse perineal muscle.

The deepest muscles are the obturator internus, coccygeus, and levator ani, made up of the puborectalis, pubococcygeus, and iliococcygeus.

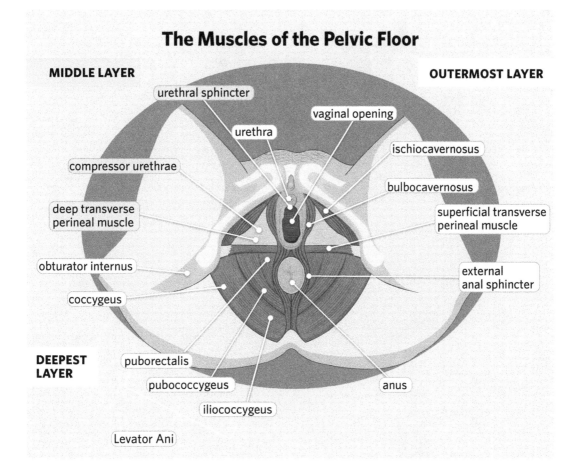

The Muscles of the Pelvic Floor

MIDDLE LAYER

OUTERMOST LAYER

urethral sphincter

vaginal opening

urethra

ischiocavernosus

compressor urethrae

bulbocavernosus

deep transverse
perineal muscle

superficial transverse
perineal muscle

obturator internus

external
anal sphincter

coccygeus

DEEPEST
LAYER

puborectalis

pubococcygeus

anus

iliococcygeus

Levator Ani

There are also muscles in the hips and buttocks that support the pelvic floor, including the piriformis, gluteus maximus, gluteus medius, gluteus minimus, and obturator internus.

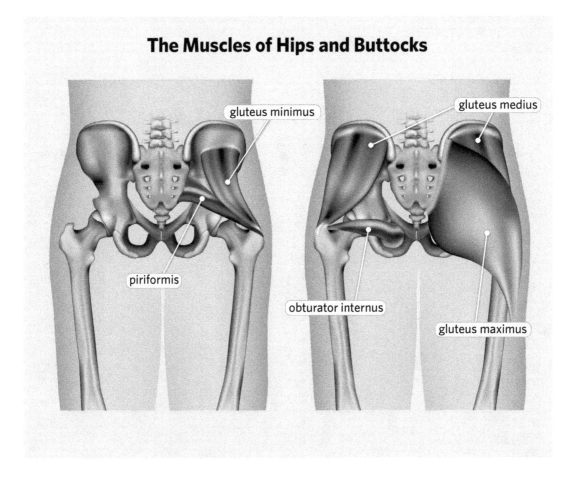

The Muscles of Hips and Buttocks

gluteus minimus

gluteus medius

piriformis

obturator internus

gluteus maximus

Although this may seem like a complicated labyrinth of muscles, just think of them as a network of muscles that can work together collectively. You don't need to memorize all the muscles and their locations, but it can be helpful to have this basic overview.

Why Pelvic Floors Can Weaken

The pelvic floor muscles can weaken over time as a result of events and circumstances, or they may simply be weak from an early age. Pregnancy, childbirth, surgery, trauma or injury, prostate cancer, menopause, aging, certain sports, intense exercise, lack of exercise, and chronic back pain are some factors that can weaken pelvic floor muscles.

Pregnancy and childbirth are two of the most common risk factors for a weak pelvic floor. Weight gain and pressure from the developing fetus can damage the muscles in the pelvis. Vaginal birth can cause trauma and further damage to the area, resulting in weakened muscles, among other symptoms. Some people may not experience any postpartum change to their pelvic floor muscles, especially if pelvic floor strengthening and stretching exercises were performed throughout pregnancy. However, sometimes injury to the area is unavoidable, and it's often unpredictable.

Many people experience one or more of these risk factors, which can lead to even more weakness in the pelvic floor muscles and may make it more difficult to rebuild and strengthen the muscles. However, working to strengthen these muscles can only help, and in doing so, you can improve your quality of life.

Signs of a Weak Pelvic Floor

When the pelvic floor muscles weaken, they can lose their tone, strength, and control. This may result in:

- Difficulty completing a bowel movement

- Difficulty during childbirth

- Difficulty emptying the bladder

- Frequent urination

- Incontinence

- Painful sex

- Pelvic pain

- Uncontrollable flatulence

Bladder control support is probably the most noticeable contribution of the pelvic floor muscles. When this group of muscles is not functioning properly, it's almost impossible to hold urine in as normal with a full bladder. Depending on the severity of the muscles' weakness, it's often necessary to empty the bladder more frequently to prevent leaks and accidents.

Naturally, these symptoms can make everyday situations unpleasant and negatively affect your mental health over time, resulting in diminished mood and self-esteem. Fortunately, there is much you can do to strengthen the pelvic floor and, subsequently, overcome these issues.

Strengthening the Pelvic Floor

Strengthening the pelvic floor muscles can be achieved in the same way you would work to strengthen any other muscle in your body. If you regularly work to engage and stretch certain muscles with specific exercises that target that muscle group, you will invariably achieve more muscle tone and control. If you have a specific issue that needs to be addressed, you can still work on strengthening and stretching the entire muscle group as a whole in order to see improvements. For example, if you just gave birth and you notice that you are having trouble controlling your bladder, you don't need to target the specific muscle in the pelvic floor that may be causing the problem. Instead, you can focus on consistently and routinely exercising the area as a whole, which will likely result in additional improvements to health and strength over time. Regular and continuous work on these muscles will ensure that improvements come more rapidly and their health is maintained for the long term.

Advantages of a Strong Pelvic Floor

A strong pelvic floor can lead to a better quality of life, due to its positive impact on both your overall physical health and mental well-being. Strengthening your pelvic muscles can have a positive impact on your sexual sensitivity and lead to improved bladder control, less overall pelvic pain, and more. Because the pelvic floor muscles are a part of your core, strengthening the pelvic floor can improve your core strength. Another advantage to strengthening the pelvic floor muscles is improved posture. The muscles in the pelvis support the hips and lower back, so if the pelvic muscles are strong, the muscles they support can function better as well. All these physical improvements can affect your mental health, leading to an increased sense of self-confidence and self-esteem. You may also experience a range of other benefits specific to you, your body, and your goals.

Understanding Kegel Exercises

Kegel exercises are named after American gynecologist Dr. Arnold Kegel, who introduced the exercises in 1948. He created these exercises to help prevent or treat conditions such as pelvic organ prolapse or incontinence. Before Dr. Kegel, ancient yogic texts discussed the use of the *mula bandha*, the Sanskrit term for "root lock," an exercise to draw up the root chakra (based in the perineum) and activate the muscles in the pelvic area.

If you have pelvic floor muscle weakness, Kegel exercises can be a good way to strengthen these muscles. The exercises are discreet, so you can do them anywhere, and they don't take much time. They can be done along with the pelvic floor yoga practices described in this book.

Unfortunately, many people may not be practicing Kegels effectively. They may be activating the muscles, but not in the specific way that the Kegel exercise requires to actually strengthen the muscles. Additionally, many people who practice Kegels should not be practicing them. If your pelvic floor muscles are tight, or if you've had surgeries or procedures that made the muscles tight, Kegel exercises are not right for you—pelvic floor release exercises are a better choice. Stretching and relaxing the area is also highly recommended for all.

Exercise: Practicing Kegels Correctly

Here is an easy way to help yourself practice Kegels effectively:

1. Visualize the muscles of the pelvic floor between the two sit bones at the bottom of your pelvis.

2. Inhale deeply through your nose. As you exhale, bring the muscles together as if you are closing a book. Then, imagine you are lifting the muscles up toward your abdomen. Hold for a moment, then release.

3. Visualize the muscles of the pelvic floor between your pubic bone and tailbone, and draw those muscles together and up in the same way. Hold for a moment, then release.

4. Now, visualize the muscles between all four corners: the two sit bones, the pubic bone, and the tailbone. Draw them all together to meet in the middle, lift them up toward your abdomen, and hold for a moment before releasing.

5. Repeat this exercise 5 to 10 times, several times a week.

The Benefits of Pelvic Floor Yoga

As mentioned earlier, yoga is extremely beneficial to health and well-being, and practicing yoga specifically for your pelvic floor is a great way to bring more health and vitality to the area. There are many types of yoga poses for the pelvic floor, and each can help strengthen, heal, energize, relax, restore, and/or harmonize the pelvic floor muscles. Poses such as the **Wide-Legged Squat** (page 30) provide a deep stretch and release for the pelvic floor muscles. Other poses, such as the **Bound Angle Pose** (page 34), help open your pelvis by increasing the external rotation of your hips and promoting hip and hamstring flexibility. Like all yoga poses, poses for the pelvic floor can help you connect your mind and body for increased self-awareness. A pelvic floor yoga practice helps create more balance within your pelvic floor and throughout your whole body. A regular pelvic floor yoga practice can help you connect with your body in a deeper way. You will feel great on the yoga mat, as well as in your everyday life.

Pelvic floor yoga can be your primary form of pelvic floor muscle exercise, or you can incorporate other types of exercise you may already be doing. For instance, if you would like to incorporate the Kegel exercises described earlier, you can do so before or after your pelvic floor yoga practice, do them on the days you do not practice pelvic floor yoga, or add them to your yoga practice. Do whatever feels most comfortable.

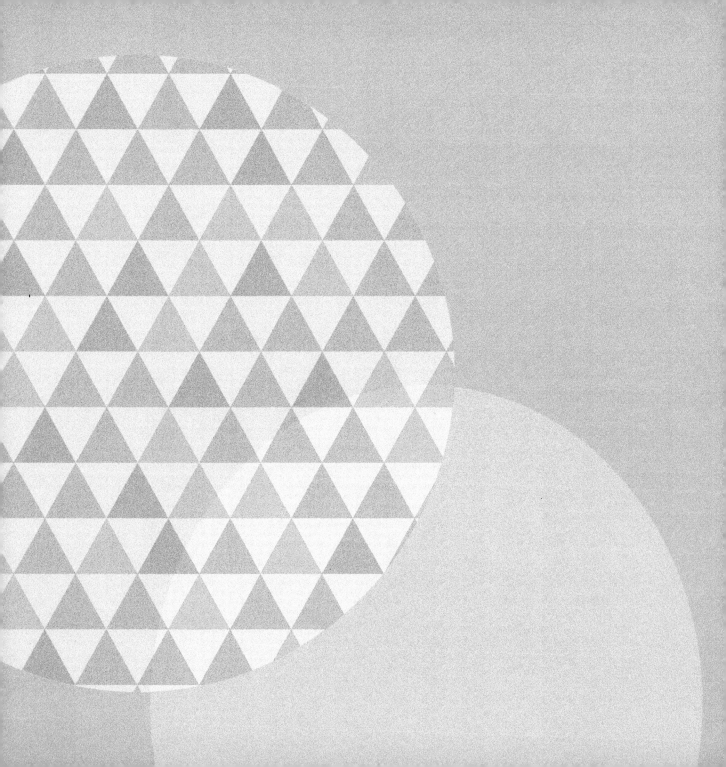

CHAPTER TWO

Preparing for Pelvic Floor Yoga

The information in this chapter will help you prepare for a successful and positive pelvic floor yoga experience. I'll share how to make the most of your yoga practice and achieve the greatest benefits, so you can witness your desired results becoming a reality in your life.

There are just a few simple steps and things you should know before jumping into a pelvic floor yoga practice—I'll share all of that with you now.

Your Yoga Essentials

Whether you are a complete beginner or an experienced yogi, there is something for yoga practitioners of all levels to learn and take away from this book. This section covers the essentials you will need to practice pelvic floor yoga at home or wherever you would like.

For starters, it is important to provide a safe space to practice your pelvic floor yoga. Having a safe and comfortable space for yourself that is dedicated to your yoga practice will help ensure a successful and pleasant pelvic floor yoga journey.

Also key to success is wearing something comfortable to practice pelvic floor yoga. It may seem trivial, but what you wear when you practice the yoga asanas makes a huge difference in how your practice goes. I'll also speak about props you may need for your yoga practice and substitutions you can use if you do not have the specified props available.

Other topics covered in this section include what to look for with pelvic floor progress, how to be mindful of how you are feeling, the importance of breath, and perhaps most important, how to make pelvic floor yoga a successful habit in your life.

A Safe Space

You can practice anywhere you like—your home, office, outdoors, or anywhere you need to—as long as you feel comfortable and have some room to move your body without obstructions. The space should be big enough to fit a yoga mat with several feet around the mat to move your arms and legs. It should also be on level ground, so you can balance without falling over. This practice space should be a somewhat quiet place, where you can focus on what you are doing. If you have others in the house with you, you may want to use earplugs or wireless headphones with soft, calming music to prevent distractions from outside noise.

You may feel guilty or stressed making time for yourself to practice yoga. Remind yourself to be compassionate and loving to yourself and grant yourself the time and space needed to heal and take care of your body and mind.

Comfortable Clothes

While practicing pelvic floor yoga, it's important to dress for the experience. Wearing clothes that are uncomfortable or restrictive can negatively impact your yoga practice in several ways. Ill-fitting clothes can distract you, causing you to focus more on the clothing than what you are meant to be doing in your yoga practice. If your clothing is too tight or restrictive, you may not be able to move freely enough to execute the yoga poses. If your clothing is too loose, you could get your limbs, hands, or feet caught in the clothing while practicing, which could cause you to trip or fall over. The proper clothing depends on you and what you are comfortable in—aim for attire that fits well and makes you feel comfortable.

Possible Props

You can practice yoga anywhere, and all you truly need is yourself and some space to move. However, there are certain props that can make your yoga experience more comfortable and accessible.

Here are some props you may find useful:

- Bolster
- Strap
- Yoga blanket
- Yoga blocks (foam, cork, or wooden)
- Yoga mat

The most important prop you'll need from this list is a yoga mat, because other alternatives, such as blankets or towels, do not provide the traction required to remain stable in some of the poses. However, you can substitute household items for the other props, if needed. The blocks can be substituted with thick books, and the blanket can be replaced with a regular blanket or thick towels. For the strap, use a sturdy scarf or belt, and for the bolster, use bed pillows.

Pelvic Floor Progress

As your yoga practice progresses, you will start to notice some positive changes in your pelvic floor and body overall. You may begin to feel stronger or less discomfort in the pelvis. You also may begin to notice some of your related symptoms start to heal and slowly improve. It all depends on where you are in your pelvic floor yoga journey and your personal circumstances. If you're pregnant and working on your pelvic floor to assist with labor, you'll have a very different experience than someone healing from surgery in the area. Improvement and progress will look different for everyone.

To ensure you are progressing, you may want to set goals and check in with yourself. Different ways to measure progress include assessing for more energy, less incontinence, increased core muscle strength, less pain, improved muscle flexibility, improved joint mobility, more confidence, improved self-esteem, and more. If your goal is to feel less pain and experience less incontinence throughout the day, after a week or two of regular practice, check in with yourself to evaluate any improvements in those areas. If you're not experiencing the desired progress, perhaps tweaking your yoga practice slightly will allow you to achieve your goals more efficiently.

Remember, yoga practice is all about consistency. The only way you will see true progress is by practicing on a regular basis. This doesn't mean you have to practice every day. It just means practicing regularly and consistently. For instance, you can practice once per week for an hour or every other day for 10 to 15 minutes, depending on your schedule and comfort level. Once you've maintained a practice for several weeks or months, you may start to see small improvements. Try not to get discouraged if you don't see changes in the amount of time you originally expected. Be patient and kind with yourself, and you will surely see the improvements you desire in the amount of time that is right for you.

Pay Attention to How You Feel

With any physical practice, it's important to check in with your body often and pay attention to how you feel. Doing so will help you avoid injury and strain and continue to heal and strengthen at a steady pace.

While practicing pelvic floor yoga, the feeling you should look for is a "lifting up" of the pelvic floor muscles and the surrounding muscles. The area should feel lighter, as if there is less pressure or tension. In certain poses, where you are in a more passive and relaxed state, you may not feel this sense of lifting up as intensely as you do in more active poses. Pay attention to how you feel as you practice, making sure you don't overwork the muscles and create an overly tight or fatigued pelvic floor.

When you begin to work your pelvic floor muscles more often and engage those muscles along with your other core muscles, you may experience a sensation of "bearing down." This means that the muscles have become overly tight, which can cause other health issues, such as more pelvic pain. If you are pregnant and preparing for a vaginal labor, this overtightening of the pelvic floor muscles can increase the risk of tearing your perineum or needing an episiotomy during labor. In fact, some people experience this type of tightness due to trauma or surgery in the area. In this case, focus more on pelvic floor release rather than strengthening the area.

Breathing Harmony Into the Pelvic Floor

The role of breath, known as *prana* in yoga, is crucial to a pelvic floor yoga practice and yoga in general. It is important to know how to breathe properly to achieve optimal health in your pelvic floor muscles while practicing yoga. It is also good to know how to coordinate your movement in yoga with your inhales and exhales. Knowing the proper way to breathe through your body while practicing yoga will help you feel energized, healthy, relaxed, and revitalized.

In yoga, prana is known as the life source and your source of power and energy. If done in the proper way, prana can help you feel better throughout your entire body, including your pelvic floor. When practicing pelvic floor yoga, you'll focus specifically on breathing through the pelvis and lower abdominals. You can do this by visualizing and feeling the pelvic floor and abdominals expanding and letting the air in as you inhale. When you exhale, you will feel the abdominal muscles contract back inward and the pelvic floor muscles lift up to release the air from the body slowly and gently.

In yoga, you're encouraged to inhale and exhale through the nose, not the mouth. These are several reasons that breathing through the nose is beneficial, but the main reason is that it filters the air more efficiently than when you breathe through your mouth.

Exercise: Connect to Your Pelvic Floor

The following exercise will allow you to practice feeling the connection between your breath, pelvic floor, and abdominal muscles. The more you practice, the better you will get at maintaining this connection throughout your entire yoga practice.

1. Lie on your back with knees bent and feet flat on the ground.

2. Place a yoga block (or book or pillow) between your knees, keeping thighs hip-width apart and parallel. Make sure there is a gap between your lower back and the ground to ensure a neutral position of the spine.

3. Close your eyes and breathe deeply in and out through your nose. Feel the pelvic floor and lower abdominals expand as you inhale, and feel them contract as you exhale. Repeat for 8 to 10 full breaths.

Making Pelvic Floor Yoga a Habit

It bears repeating that to see results and improvements in your pelvic floor muscles and overall health, it is important to practice yoga regularly and consistently. Over time, you will see the results that you have set as goals for yourself. Being kind, gentle, and patient with yourself is key to enjoying the process and achieving positive results.

You don't have to practice yoga for hours every day to begin seeing the kind of results you want. Just make sure you practice regularly and consistently. Simply spend 10 minutes every other day practicing a few short pelvic floor yoga sequences. If you have longer periods of available time but only once or twice a week, then consider practicing for an hour to an hour and a half once a week. These are just examples—customize your practice to fit your schedule and lifestyle. Your practice doesn't even have to be on the same day or at the same times every week—as long as you practice, you will see results.

It's also important to set goals for yourself. Ask yourself, *What do I want to achieve with my pelvic floor yoga practice?* Set small and measurable goals for yourself that you can work toward. Smaller goals are more helpful because they're easier to reach, and once you reach them, you build your self-confidence to achieve the next goal.

PART II

PELVIC FLOOR YOGA POSES AND SEQUENCES

It's time to get started! In part 2, we'll cover specific yoga poses and instructions on how to practice them. Each pose is designed for a different purpose: healing, energizing, or harmonizing your pelvic floor muscles. You'll then find these poses in the 10 yoga sequences provided, each having a specific pelvic floor theme or purpose. By engaging in both individual poses and yoga sequences, you'll have the tools and information to create a customized pelvic floor yoga practice that is right for you.

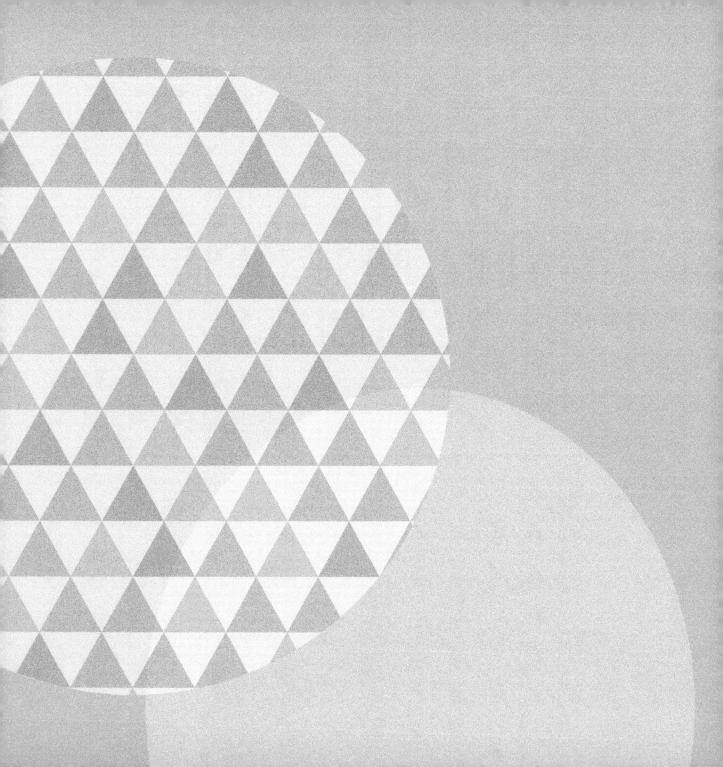

CHAPTER THREE

Healing Poses for the Pelvic Floor

In this chapter, I share yoga poses that promote healing of the pelvic floor muscles. These poses are great for anyone to practice, even if you have experienced trauma or surgery in the area. If the area is overly tight and in need of a stretch, these poses can really help. These poses are meant to help you recover from the stress of trauma or surgery, loss of muscle tone, loss of control, or any other pelvic floor muscle issues.

Child's Pose: Balasana

BENEFITS: Promotes hip and hamstring flexibility, induces relaxation and calm

PRECAUTIONS: Use caution or avoid this pose if you have recently suffered an injury or have chronic pain in your knees, hamstrings, hips, or back. Skip if you cannot place weight on your feet or ankles.

INSTRUCTIONS:

1. Come onto your hands and knees into a tabletop position, keeping your hands and arms under your shoulders, with your knees hip-width apart.

2. Touch your big toes together and separate your knees slightly wider than your rib cage.

3. Sit onto your heels and rest your torso on top of your thighs. Bring your forehead to the ground.

4. Reach your arms out in front of you, placing your palms flat on the floor.

5. Breathe deeply, expanding your ribcage and your pelvic floor muscles with each inhale.

6. With each exhale, feel the ribs coming back inward and the pelvic floor lifting upward.

7. Continue for 8 to 10 full breaths.

8. To come out of the pose, simply bring your torso back up to a seated position on your heels.

TIP: If you experience joint pain in this pose, place a rolled blanket behind your knees and place a block, pillow, or folded blanket under your forehead on the ground.

Happy Baby: Ananda Balasana

BENEFITS: Promotes hip and hamstring flexibility, releases pelvic floor muscles

PRECAUTIONS: Use caution or avoid this pose if you have recently suffered an injury or have chronic pain in your hips, knees, hamstrings, or lower back.

INSTRUCTIONS:

1. Lie flat on your back with your knees bent and feet on the ground, keeping your spine neutral.

2. Bring your knees up toward your chest.

3. Keeping your legs separate, grab onto the pinky toe-sides of your feet with your hands while flexing both feet.

4. Lift your legs so the bottoms of your feet are facing the ceiling and your knees are in toward your armpits. You should feel a rather deep stretch in the hamstrings.

5. Hold here for 8 to 10 full breaths.

6. To come out of this pose, release your hands from your feet and bring your knees back in toward the chest, then slowly place your legs back down on the ground.

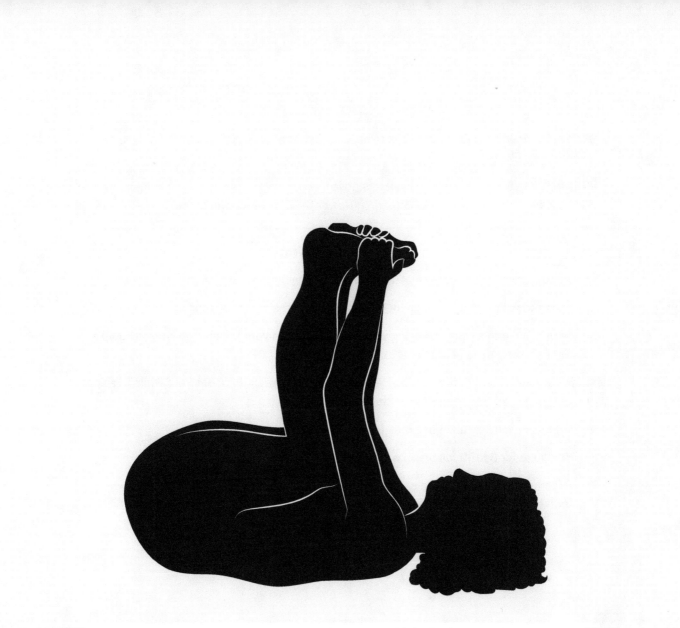

TIP: If you cannot reach your feet in this pose, hold the back of your thighs instead.

Wide-Legged Squat: Malasana

BENEFITS: Provides deep stretch and release for pelvic floor muscles, promotes hip and hamstring flexibility

PRECAUTIONS: Use caution or avoid this pose if you have recently suffered an injury or have chronic pain in your hips, knees, hamstrings, lower back, ankles, or feet.

INSTRUCTIONS:

1. Stand with your feet about mat-width apart. Face your toes outward at an angle.

2. Bring the palms of your hands together to meet at the center of your chest.

3. Bend down into a squat, bringing your hips lower than your knees. The knees should not come forward beyond the big toes.

4. Bring your elbows to the inside of your knees to help keep them outward while keeping your hands at the center of your chest.

5. Keep your spine straight and look forward.

6. Hold here for 8 to 10 full breaths.

7. To come out of this pose, release your hands, bringing them to the floor, and slowly help yourself to a standing position.

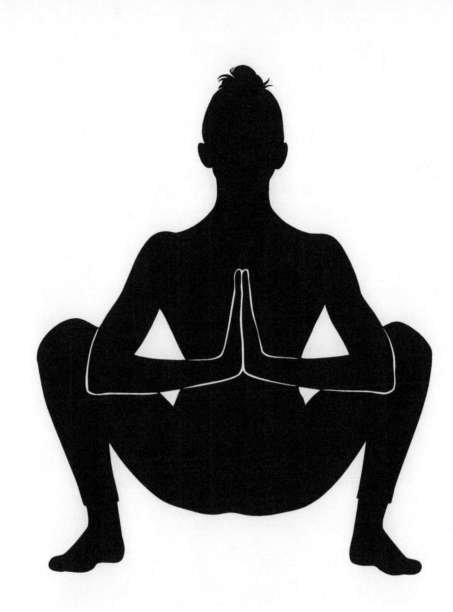

 TIP: If this pose feels too intense for your pelvic floor or hip muscles, sit on a yoga block, bolster, or folded blanket.

Easy Pose: Sukhasana

BENEFITS: Promotes mindfulness, induces relaxation, relaxes and releases pelvic floor muscles

PRECAUTIONS: Use caution or avoid this pose if you have recently suffered an injury or have chronic pain in your knees, hips, hamstrings, or back.

INSTRUCTIONS:

1. Come to a seated position on the ground.

2. Cross your shins, bringing your right leg in front of your left.

3. Flex both feet, bringing them under your knees.

4. Sit up tall, straightening your spine, and bring your hands to your knees.

5. Close your eyes and meditate here, if you'd like.

6. Breathe deeply in and out through your nose.

7. Hold this pose as long as you want.

8. Release your hands from your knees, uncross your shins, cross them in the opposite direction, and repeat the pose on the other side to maintain symmetry.

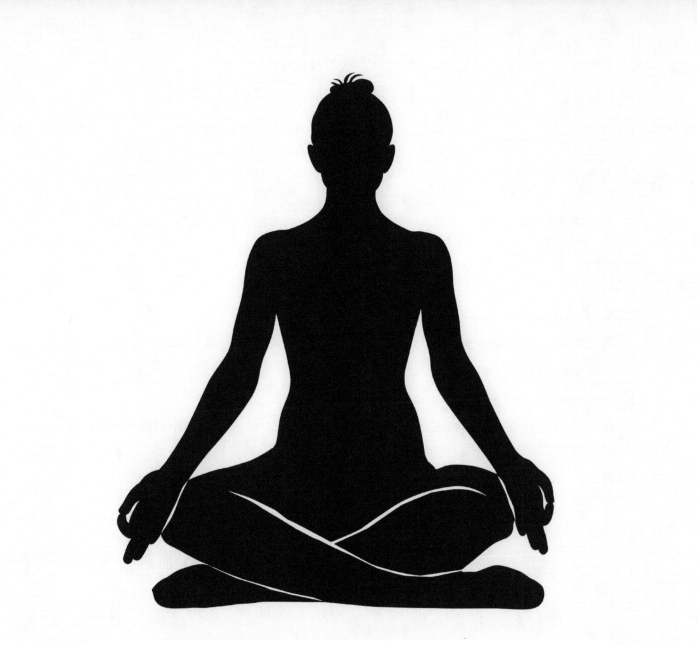

TIP: To ease joint pain in this pose, sit on a folded blanket.

Bound Angle Pose: Baddha Konasana

BENEFITS: Increases external rotation of the hips, promotes overall hip flexibility, releases pelvic floor muscles

PRECAUTIONS: Use caution or avoid this pose if you have recently suffered an injury or have chronic pain in your knees, hips, or hamstrings.

INSTRUCTIONS:

1. Come to a seated position on the ground.

2. Bring the bottoms of your feet to meet each other and keep your knees out to the side.

3. Hold on to your feet with your hands and sit up tall.

4. Hold here for 8 to 10 full breaths.

5. To come out of this pose, release your hands from your feet, bring your knees back in toward each other, and straighten your legs.

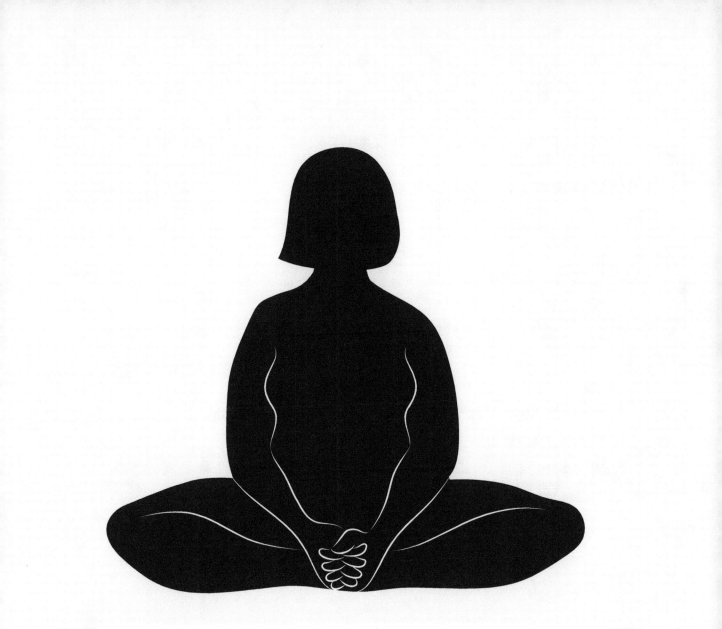

TIP: If you experience lower back pain in this pose, sit on a folded blanket to relieve some of the pressure.

Low Lunge: Anjaneyasana

BENEFITS: Improves balance, promotes hamstring flexibility, stretches surrounding muscles of the pelvic floor

PRECAUTIONS: Use caution or avoid this pose if you have recently suffered an injury or have chronic pain in your legs, hips, hamstrings, feet, or ankles.

INSTRUCTIONS:

1. Come onto your hands and knees into a tabletop position, keeping your hands and arms under your shoulders, with your knees hip-width apart.

2. Bring your right leg forward, between your hands, and keep your toes facing forward and your knee directly above your ankle. Your left knee should be on the ground, and you should feel a stretch in the front of your left thigh. You should also feel a deep stretch in the right hip socket, as well as a lengthening of your left hip joint.

3. Look down toward the ground, keeping length in your spine and neck.

4. Hold here for 8 to 10 full breaths.

5. To come out of this pose, bring your right knee back underneath your hips.

6. Repeat on the other side.

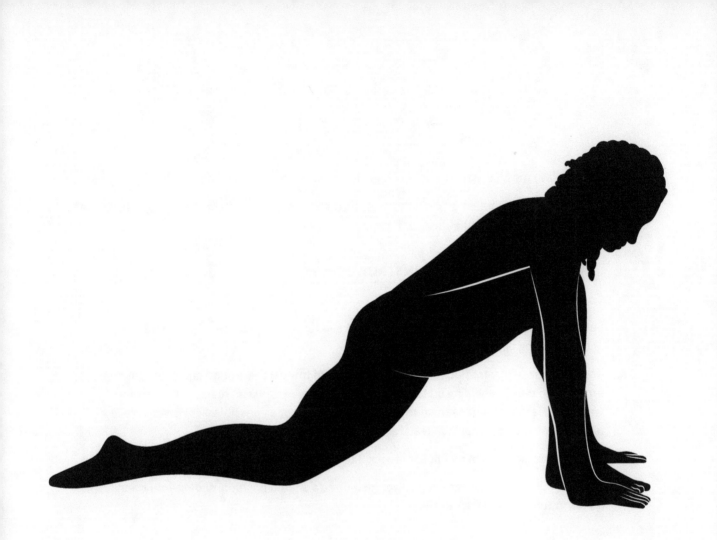

 TIP: If you feel knee pain when you place your knee on the ground, fold your yoga mat over, so you have extra cushioning underneath your knee.

Seated Wide-Legged Forward Fold: Upavistha Konasana

BENEFITS: Promotes hip, hamstring, and back flexibility, releases pelvic floor muscles

PRECAUTIONS: Use caution or avoid this pose if you have recently suffered an injury or have chronic pain in your hips, hamstrings, or back.

INSTRUCTIONS:

1. Come to a seated position on the ground.

2. Spread both legs out to the sides in a wide V, keeping your legs straight and your knees and toes facing up toward the ceiling.

3. Keeping your spine straight, fold your torso forward toward the ground and place your arms out to the side holding on to your feet. Alternatively, you can reach both arms forward and place your forehead on the floor or as close to it as possible. Feel free to place a folded blanket under your forehead for support.

4. Keep your spine straight and hold here for 8 to 10 deep breaths.

5. To come out of this pose, gently pull yourself up to a seated position, sliding your hands on the ground toward your pelvis.

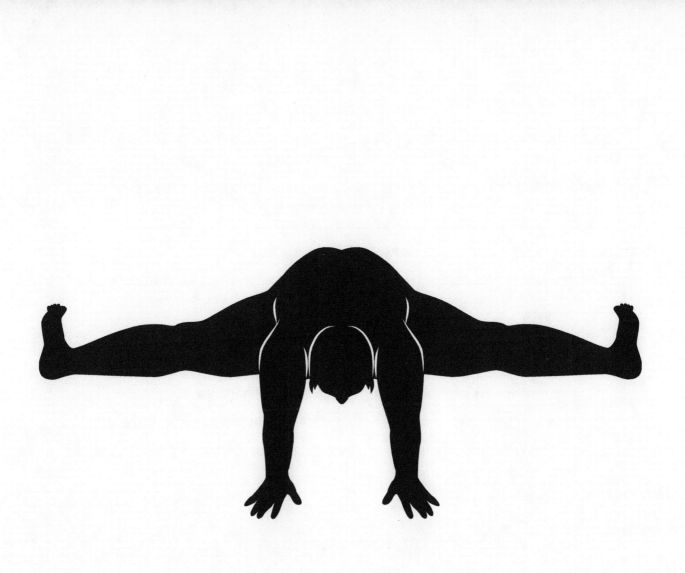

TIP: Bring the legs in closer to each other if you can't keep both legs straight and the knees and toes facing the ceiling.

Cat/Cow: Marjariasana/Bitilasana

BENEFITS: Promotes mobility in the spine and neck, gently lubricates the joints in the hips and pelvis

PRECAUTIONS: Use caution or avoid this pose if you have recently suffered an injury or have chronic pain in your knees, hands, wrists, shoulders, neck, or back.

INSTRUCTIONS:

1. Come onto your hands and knees into a tabletop position, keeping your hands and arms under your shoulders, with your knees hip-width apart. Keep your spine neutral.

2. On your inhale, arch your back in, looking up and forward, and spreading your shoulders wide apart into cow pose.

3. On your exhale, curve your spine upward in the opposite direction, feeling it reach up toward the ceiling. Look downward toward your thighs with your gaze.

4. Continue with this pattern of breath and movement for 8 to 10 repetitions.

5. To complete this sequence, bring your spine back into a neutral position.

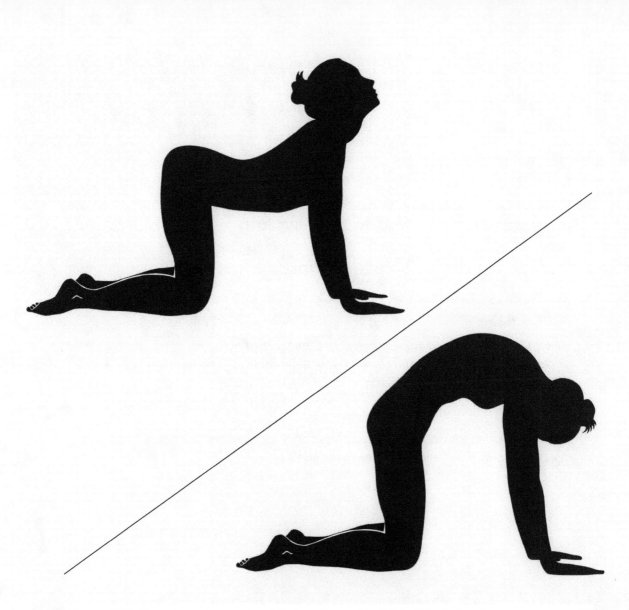

TIP: If you have knee pain while kneeling, add a folded blanket under your knees for extra cushioning and support.

Melting Heart/Puppy Pose: Uttana Shishosana

BENEFITS: Stretches the back, hips, and hamstrings, releases and stretches the pelvic floor muscles

PRECAUTIONS: Use caution or avoid this pose if you have recently suffered an injury or have chronic pain in your back, knees, shoulders, hips, or hamstrings.

INSTRUCTIONS:

1. Come onto your hands and knees into a tabletop position, keeping your hands and arms under your shoulders, with your knees hip-width apart.

2. Reach your arms forward and bring your forehead to the floor, keeping the backside lifted and staying on your knees. You can keep your spine straight or come into a slight arch for a deeper chest and shoulder stretch.

3. Hold here for 8 to 10 deep breaths.

4. To come out of this pose, gently lift your head off the ground and bring your chest back up, coming onto your hands and knees back into a tabletop position.

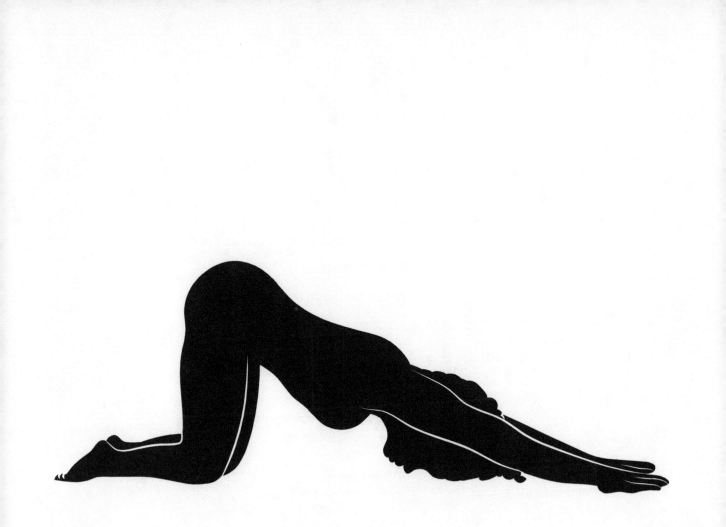

 TIP: Place a folded blanket under your head and arms to alleviate any pressure in your hips, spine, and/or shoulders.

Reclined Pigeon Pose: Supta Kapotasana

BENEFITS: Promotes hip and hamstring flexibility, releases pelvic floor muscles

PRECAUTIONS: Use caution or avoid this pose if you have recently suffered an injury or have chronic pain in your hips, hamstrings, or lower back.

INSTRUCTIONS:

1. Lie on your back with your knees bent and feet flat on the floor.

2. Keep your left foot on the floor and your knee pointing up while you hug the right knee in toward your chest.

3. Turn the right leg out from the hip and cross the right ankle over your left thigh.

4. Bring your right hand in between your legs and hold on to your left hamstrings with both hands. Bring both legs in this shape toward your chest, keeping your feet flexed.

5. Hold here and breathe for 8 to 10 full breaths.

6. To come out of this pose, slowly release your hands from your leg and bring both legs down toward the ground. Uncross your ankle from your thigh.

7. Repeat on the other side.

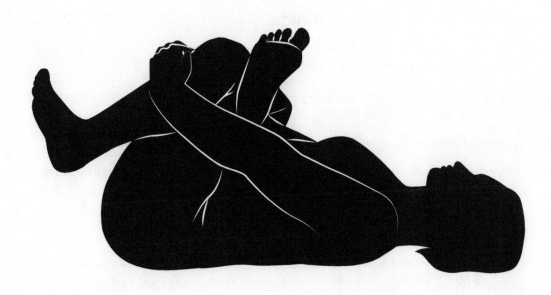

 TIP: If you cannot reach behind your leg to hold your thigh in this pose, use a yoga strap to wrap around it and hold on to instead.

High Lunge: Ashta Chandrasana

BENEFITS: Energizes the body, strengthens the legs and pelvic floor muscles

PRECAUTIONS: Use caution or avoid doing this pose if you have recently suffered an injury or have chronic pain in your ankles, legs, knees, hips, back, or shoulders.

INSTRUCTIONS:

1. Come onto your hands and knees into a tabletop position, keeping your hands and arms under your shoulders, with your knees hip-width apart.

2. Bring your right leg forward in between your hands, keeping your toes facing forward and your knee directly above your ankle.

3. Tuck the left toes under and straighten the left leg to lift your knee off the ground.

4. Engage both leg muscles and ground them into the floor as you lift your torso and reach your arms up toward the ceiling.

5. Keeping your spine straight and your gaze looking forward, hold here for 8 to 10 full breaths.

6. To come out of this pose, bring your hands back down to the ground on either side of your right foot. Place the left knee on the ground and untuck the toes. Bring your right knee back under your body, coming back into the tabletop position.

7. Repeat on the other side.

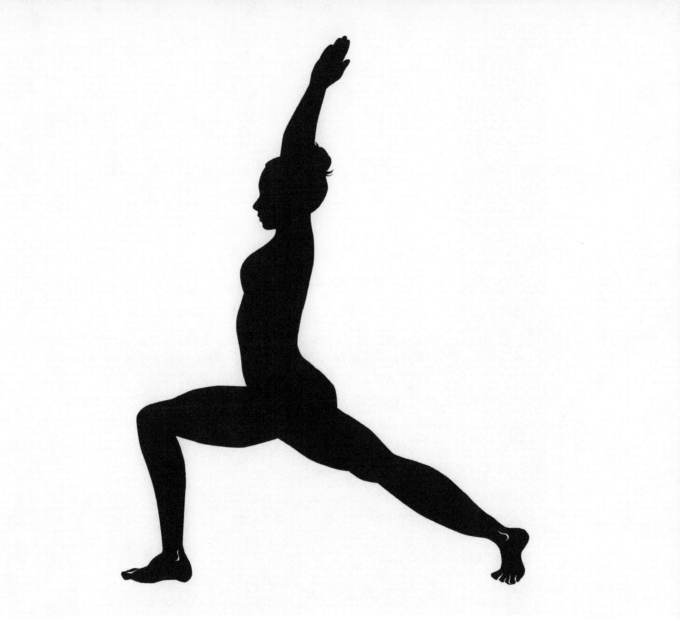

TIP: Clasp your hands together above your head and come into a slight upper back arch to give yourself more of a revitalizing energy boost.

Standing Wide-Legged Forward Fold: Prasarita Padottanasana

BENEFITS: Stretches the hips and hamstrings, releases tension in the head, neck, and pelvic floor muscles

PRECAUTIONS: Use caution or avoid this pose if you have recently suffered an injury or have chronic pain in your hips, hamstrings, back, or neck.

INSTRUCTIONS:

1. Start by standing evenly on both feet. Slowly bring your feet out to a wide stance, about the width of the length of your leg.

2. Place your hands on your hips and begin to fold your torso forward gently, then place the palms of your hands flat on the ground in line with your feet and with your fingertips pointing forward.

3. Release your head and neck muscles, allowing your head to hang freely toward the ground.

4. Hold here for 8 to 10 deep breaths.

5. To come out of this pose, bend your knees and bring your hands back to your hips. Come back up to standing with a straight spine, and bring your feet back under your hips.

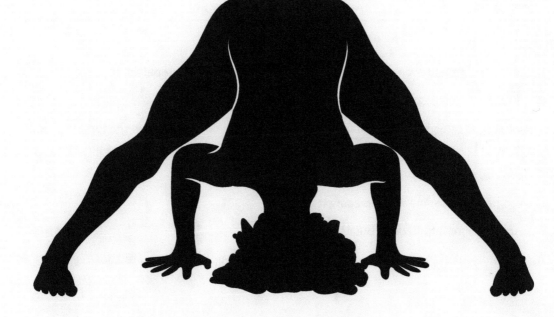

TIP: If you cannot reach the ground in this pose, place your hands on top of blocks to keep from overly rounding your spine, and bend both knees as much as you need to feel comfortable in this pose.

Straight-Legged Seated Forward Fold: Dandasana

BENEFITS: Increases hamstring flexibility, produces a calming response in your body, releases surrounding muscles of the pelvic floor

PRECAUTIONS: Use caution or avoid this pose if you have recently suffered an injury or have chronic pain in your hamstrings, tailbone, or back.

INSTRUCTIONS:

1. Sit on the ground evenly on both sit bones at the bottom of your pelvis.

2. Straighten your legs and flex both feet, keeping the toes facing up.

3. Inhale and straighten your spine, sitting up taller. On your exhale, fold the torso over and hold on to the feet, ankles, or shins with both hands.

4. Look down toward your legs with your gaze.

5. Lengthen your spine while keeping it neutral.

6. Hold here for 8 to 10 deep breaths.

7. To come out of this pose, slowly bring the torso back upright to a seated position.

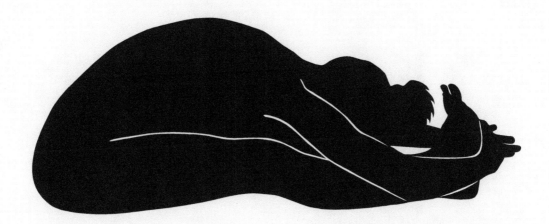

 TIP: If you are overly rounding your spine or feel lower back pain in this pose, sit on top of a folded blanket to tilt your pelvis forward.

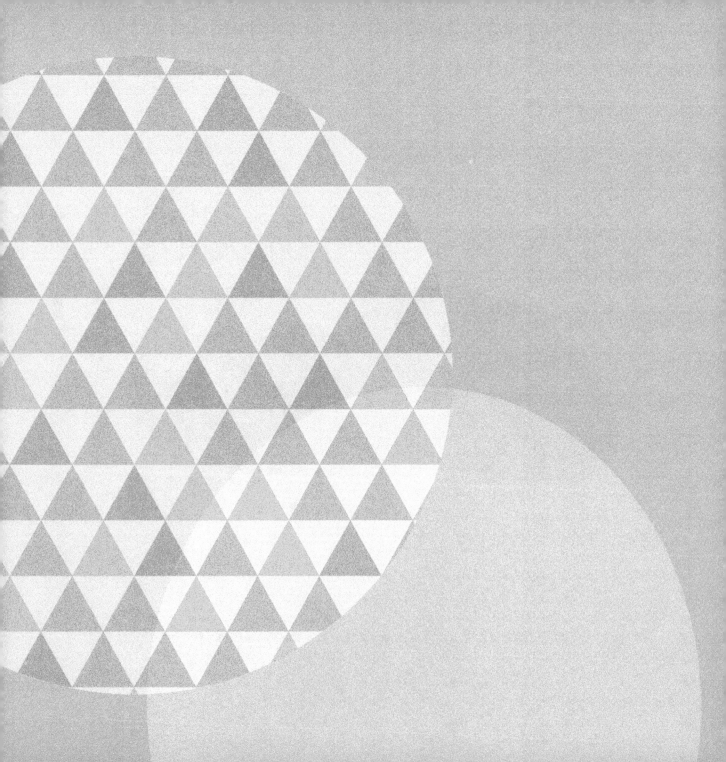

CHAPTER FOUR

Energizing Poses for the Pelvic Floor

In this chapter, we'll explore pelvic floor yoga poses to energize, strengthen, and make the pelvic floor more responsive when activated. If you have a weak pelvic floor and need to strengthen and tighten things up, these poses are the answer. If you practice these regularly and incorporate them into your yoga practice, you'll notice and feel the pelvic floor muscles getting stronger.

Mountain Pose: Tadasana

BENEFITS: Stabilizes and grounds the pelvic floor to build a solid foundation

PRECAUTIONS: Use caution or avoid this pose if you have recently suffered an injury or have chronic pain in your legs, ankles, back, or neck.

INSTRUCTIONS:

1. Stand evenly on both legs with your feet parallel and toes facing straight ahead.

2. Keep both legs straight and engage the muscles in the front of your thighs to bring the kneecaps in.

3. Keep your spine in a neutral position and look straight ahead.

4. Spread your shoulders and collarbones apart from each other, but avoid arching your back by keeping your core engaged.

5. Place your arms down by your sides with your palms facing your body. Keep your hands and fingers engaged.

6. As you hold this pose, stretch up through the crown of your head, and at the same time, dig your heels down into the ground.

7. Hold for 8 to 10 full breaths.

8. To come out of this pose, simply release.

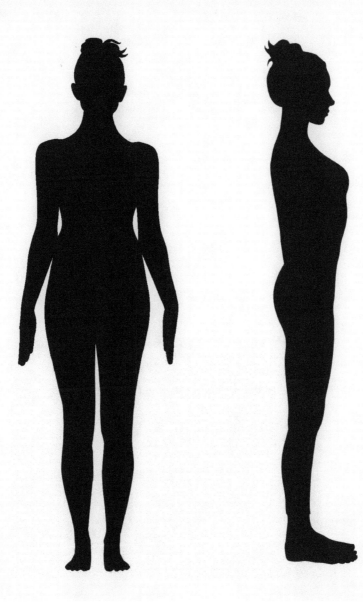

TIP: To add a stretching element to this pose, reach your arms up above your head with palms facing one another and look up toward your hands.

Downward-Facing Dog: Adho Mukha Svanasana

BENEFITS: Strengthens and stretches the pelvic floor muscles

PRECAUTIONS: Use caution or avoid this pose if you have recently suffered an injury or have chronic pain in your wrists, legs, ankles, back, or neck.

INSTRUCTIONS:

1. Come onto your hands and knees into a tabletop position, keeping your hands and arms under your shoulders with palms flat on the ground and fingers spread apart, with your knees hip-width apart.

2. Tuck your toes, press into the ground with your hands and feet, and straighten your legs while lifting your hips up.

3. Press your heels down toward the ground; it is fine if they are slightly elevated.

4. Keep your legs straight and sit bones reaching upward.

5. Let your head relax and hang freely.

6. Hold this pose for 8 to 10 full breaths.

7. To come out of this pose, gently bring your knees back down onto the ground, coming back into the tabletop position.

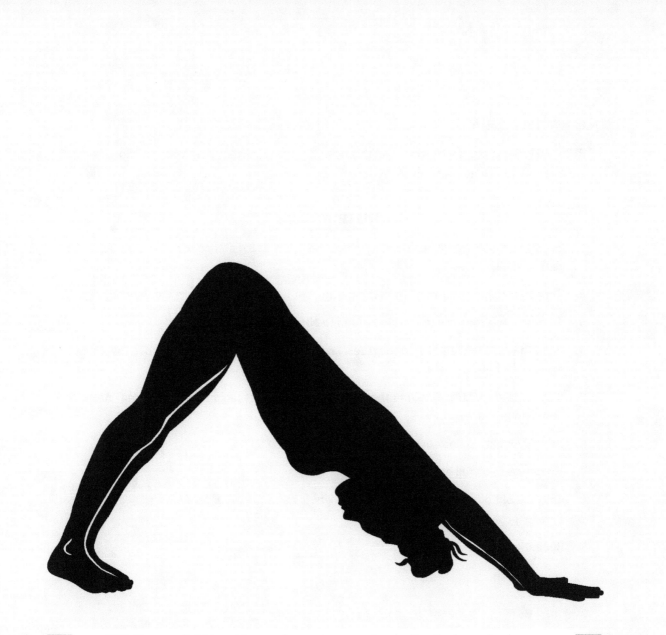

TIP: Keep a slight bend in your knees to prevent rounding the lower back.

Warrior 2: Virabhadrasana 2

BENEFITS: Strengthens the legs and pelvic floor muscles, builds confidence

PRECAUTIONS: Use caution or avoid this pose if you have recently suffered an injury or have chronic pain in your legs or ankles.

INSTRUCTIONS:

1. Begin in a wide-legged position with your feet apart at a distance of one of your legs, with feet parallel.

2. Turn your right leg outward from the hip so your toes face away from the opposite leg.

3. Turn your left toes inward on the ground to about a 45-degree angle.

4. Bend the right leg to about 90 degrees, keeping the right knee directly above the ankle. Keep the left leg straight.

5. Bring your arms straight out to the sides with your palms facing down, keeping energy in your hands and fingers.

6. Bring your gaze to look over the right arm.

7. Hold for 8 to 10 full breaths.

8. To come out of this pose, straighten the right leg and turn your feet back to a parallel position.

9. Repeat on the other side.

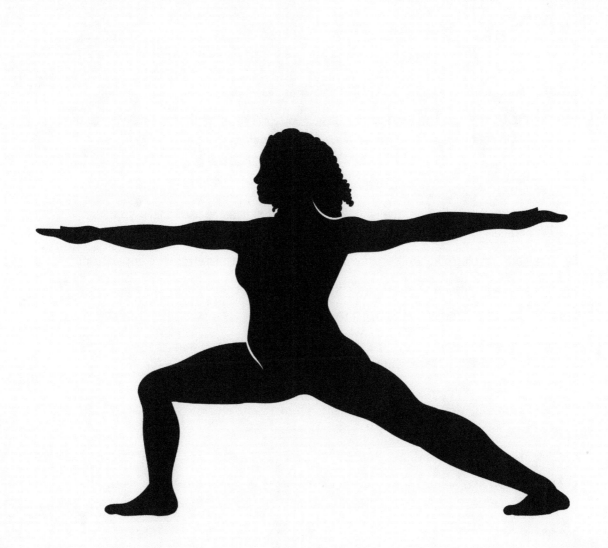

TIP: To add movement to this pose, inhale and straighten the bent leg while reaching both arms up, then return to the pose on your exhale. Repeat the cycle 10 to 15 times.

Triangle Pose: Trikonasana

BENEFITS: Strengthens the legs and pelvic floor muscles, energizes the body

PRECAUTIONS: Use caution or avoid this pose if you have recently suffered an injury or have chronic pain in your legs, ankles, hips, knees, arms, or shoulders.

INSTRUCTIONS:

1. Begin in a wide-legged position with your feet apart at a distance of one of your legs, with feet parallel.

2. Turn your right leg outward from the hip so your toes face away from the opposite leg.

3. Turn your left toes inward on the ground to about a 45-degree angle.

4. Bring your arms straight out to the sides and keep your palms facing the ground.

5. Reach your right arm over your right leg, bringing the torso over and down, keeping length in your spine. Place your hand on the ground by your foot or on top of your shin or ankle.

6. Once your right arm is stable, reach your left arm upward and look up toward the left arm if your balance permits.

7. Hold for 8 to 10 full breaths.

8. To come out of this pose, press your feet into the ground while slowly and gently lifting your torso back up and bringing your feet back to a parallel position.

9. Repeat on the other side.

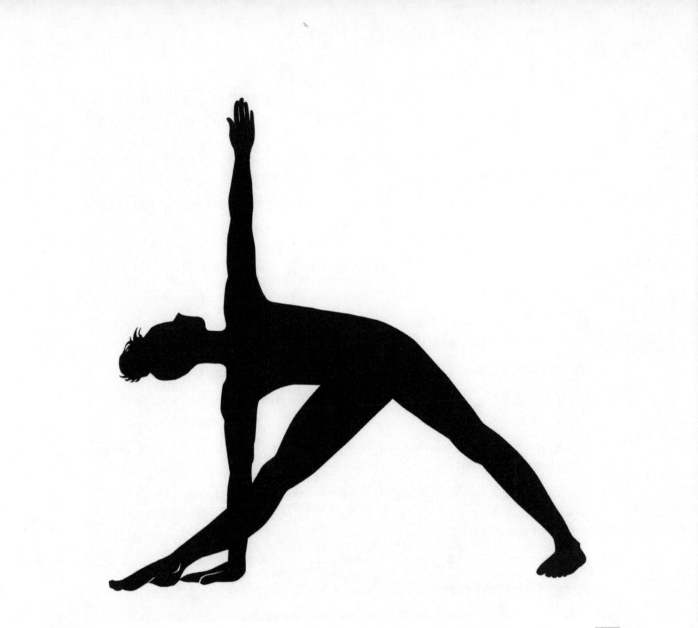

TIP: Place your hand on a yoga block (or stacked yoga blocks) if it does not touch the ground or you feel discomfort placing your hand on your leg.

Side-Angle Pose:
Utthita Parsvakonasana

BENEFITS: Strengthens the legs, trunk, and pelvic floor muscles

PRECAUTIONS: Use caution or avoid this pose if you have recently suffered an injury or have chronic pain in your legs, ankles, arms, or shoulders.

INSTRUCTIONS:

1. Begin in a wide-legged position with your feet apart at a distance of one of your legs, with feet parallel.

2. Turn your right leg outward from the hip so your toes face away from the opposite leg.

3. Turn your left toes inward on the ground to about a 45-degree angle.

4. Bend your right leg to about 90 degrees, keeping the right knee directly above the ankle. Keep the left leg straight.

5. Bring your arms straight out to the sides with your palms facing down, keeping energy in your hands and fingers.

6. Reach your right arm over your right leg, bringing the torso over and down, keeping length in your spine. Place your hand on the ground by your foot, or place your forearm on top of your right thigh.

7. Reach your left arm on a diagonal over your left ear and look upward.

8. Hold for 8 to 10 full breaths.

9. To come out of this pose, press into the ground with your feet while lifting your torso back upright. Straighten your right leg and bring the feet back to a parallel position.

10. Repeat on the other side.

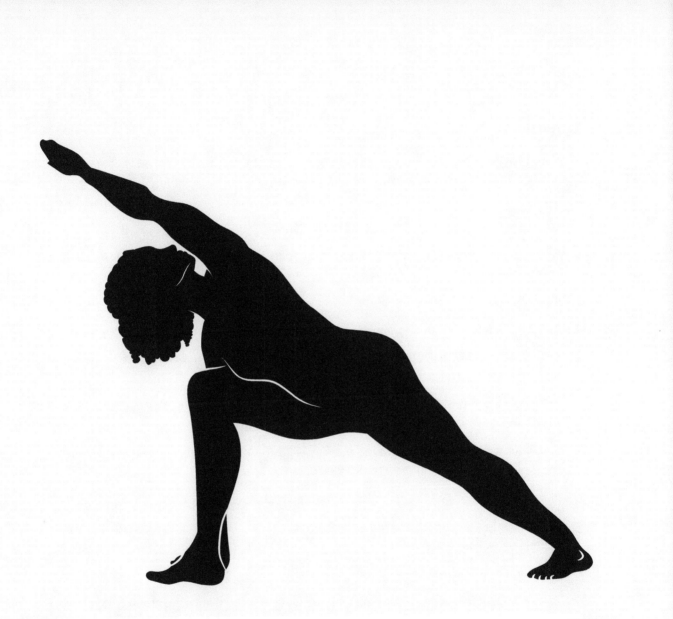

TIP: Place your hand on a yoga block (or stacked yoga blocks) if it does not touch the ground or you feel discomfort placing your forearm on your thigh.

Half-Moon Pose: Ardha Chandrasana

BENEFITS: Strengthens the leg and pelvic floor muscles, improves balance

PRECAUTIONS: Use caution or avoid this pose if you have recently suffered an injury or have chronic pain in your legs, ankles, feet, arms, or shoulders.

INSTRUCTIONS:

1. Begin in a wide-legged position with your feet apart at a distance of one of your legs, with feet parallel.

2. Turn your right leg outward from the hip so your toes face away from the opposite leg.

3. Turn your left toes inward on the ground to about a 45-degree angle.

4. Bend your right leg to about 90 degrees, keeping the right knee directly above the ankle. Keep the left leg straight.

5. Bring your arms straight out to the sides with palms facing down, keeping energy in your hands and fingers. Bring your gaze to look over your right arm.

6. Shift your weight onto your right leg and slowly lift the left leg up, bringing it parallel to the ground or higher, with the left foot flexed.

7. Place your right hand on the ground in front of your right foot, keeping it under your shoulder.

8. Reach your left arm up toward the ceiling. You can look down, straight ahead, or upward, depending on your balance.

9. Hold for 8 to 10 full breaths.

10. To come out of this pose, gently place the left foot back down onto the ground, come back through **Warrior 2** (page 58), and straighten your right leg, bringing the feet back to a parallel position.

11. Repeat on the other side.

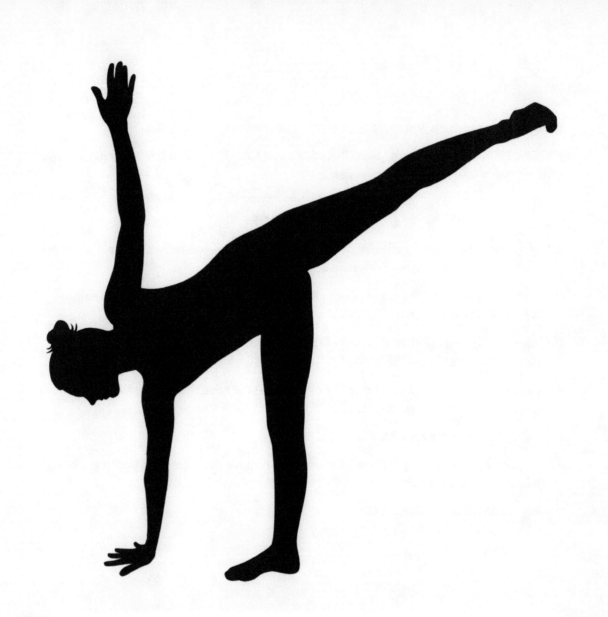

TIP: Place your bottom hand on a yoga block (or stacked yoga blocks) if it does not reach the ground.

Tree Pose: Vrksasana

BENEFITS: Strengthens and energizes the pelvic floor muscles, improves balance

PRECAUTIONS: Use caution or avoid this pose if you have recently suffered an injury or have chronic pain in your legs, ankles, or knees.

INSTRUCTIONS:

1. Stand up tall with your legs straight and feet evenly on the ground, with the big toe-sides of your feet meeting at the centerline of your body.

2. Shift your weight onto your left leg and lift your right foot off the ground. Grab hold of your shin with both hands.

3. Turn the right leg out from the hip, hold on to your ankle, and place the bottom of your right foot on the inner thigh of your left leg.

4. Bring your hands to meet at the center of your chest or raise them up straight above your head with palms facing each other.

5. Hold for 12 to 18 full breaths.

6. To come out of this pose, release your arms and remove your foot from your leg, placing it back down onto the floor.

7. Repeat on the other side.

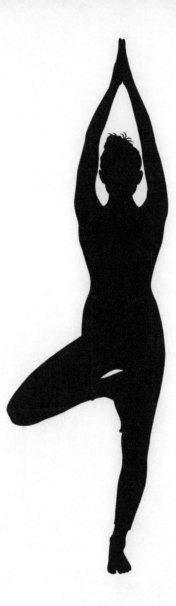

TIP: If you have trouble with balance, hold on to a wall or the back of a chair. If you have trouble with flexibility, place your foot on the bottom half of your leg instead. Do not place the foot on the knee.

Eagle Pose: Garudasana

BENEFITS: Improves hip flexibility and balance, makes the pelvic floor feel secure

PRECAUTIONS: Use caution or avoid this pose if you have recently suffered an injury or have chronic pain in your legs, ankles, hips, arms, shoulders, or knees.

INSTRUCTIONS:

1. Stand up tall with your legs straight and feet evenly on the ground, with the big toe-sides of your feet meeting at the centerline of your body.

2. Shift your weight onto your left leg and lift your right foot off the ground with your foot flexed, and cross it over the left leg in front of your body.

3. Bend the left leg into a slight squat, and with the right leg crossed over, wrap the right foot around the back of your left calf.

4. With your arms in front of you, cross the right arm over top of the left arm, and wrap your forearms around each other, so the palms of your hands meet in front of your face.

5. As you hold this the pose, look forward, and stretch through the crown of your head and your fingertips.

6. Hold for 12 to 18 full breaths.

7. To come out of the pose, release your legs and bring the right foot back down. Release your arms and place them back down by your sides.

8. Repeat on the other side.

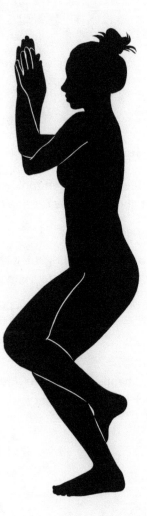

TIP: If you can't wrap your foot around your calf, place it on a block at the outer side of your left leg for stability. You can also place the backs of your hands to meet each other instead of the palms, if flexibility is an issue.

Warrior 1: Virabhadrasana 1

BENEFITS: Builds leg muscle strength, grounds the pelvic floor

PRECAUTIONS: Use caution or avoid this pose if you have recently suffered an injury or have chronic pain in your legs, ankles, or knees.

INSTRUCTIONS:

1. Begin by standing evenly on both feet. Step your left foot back about the distance of your own leg. Your left foot should be at about a 45-degree angle with your leg straight.

2. Bend your right leg to about 90 degrees.

3. Keep the hip bones facing slightly away from the right leg and turn the shoulders forward over the right knee. This should bring your torso into a very slight twist.

4. Reach your arms straight up above your head with palms facing each other. Look up with your gaze.

5. Hold for 8 to 10 full breaths.

6. To come out of this pose, place your hands on your hips, press into the ground with your right leg, and bring the left foot back to meet the right foot.

7. Repeat on the other side.

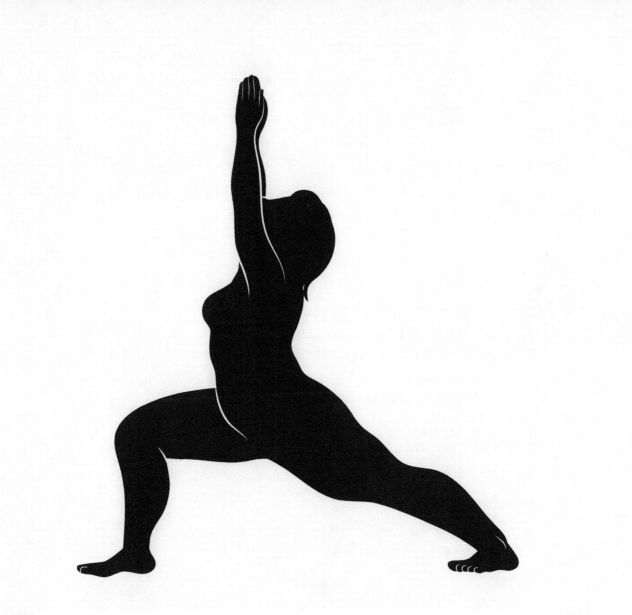

TIP: Don't get discouraged if you have trouble facing your shoulders all the way forward. It may take a while to build the flexibility to achieve this goal.

King Pigeon Pose: Eka Pada Rajakapotasana

BENEFITS: Stretches the legs and pelvic floor muscles, increasing flexibility in those areas

PRECAUTIONS: Use caution or avoid this pose if you have recently suffered an injury or have chronic pain in your legs, hips, arms, or wrists.

INSTRUCTIONS:

1. Come down onto your hands and knees and step your right leg forward in between your hands to come to a lunge position.

2. Place your hands flat on the ground at each side of your body to support your weight as you bring your pelvis toward the ground.

3. As you lower yourself, turn your right leg out from the hip and place the pinky toe-side of the leg and foot on the ground with the leg bent. Bring the right foot in line with your left hip.

4. Make sure your left knee and the top of your left foot are touching the ground.

5. Use your hands for support as you look forward, keeping length in your spine.

6. Hold for 8 to 10 full breaths.

7. To come out of this pose, press into the ground with your hands to lift your pelvis up. Tuck your left toes and bring your leg back under your pelvis.

8. Repeat on the other side.

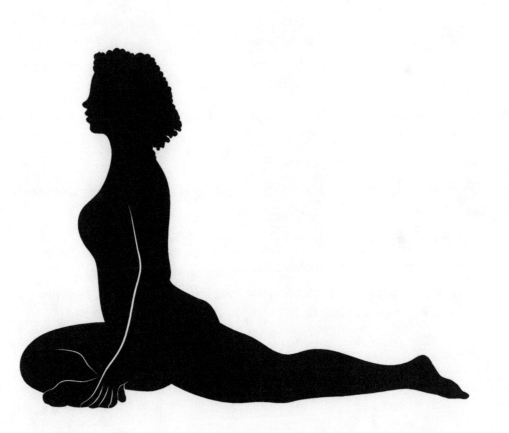

TIP: If your pelvis cannot reach the ground in this pose, use a stack of yoga blocks, folded blankets, or a yoga bolster to support your pelvis. As your flexibility increases with practice, eventually you will be able to bring your support closer and closer to the ground until it can be fully removed.

Goddess Pose: Utkata Konasana

BENEFITS: Strengthens the legs, stretches and releases the pelvic floor, builds confidence

PRECAUTIONS: Use caution or avoid this pose if you have recently suffered an injury or have chronic pain in your legs, ankles, hips, or knees.

INSTRUCTIONS:

1. Begin in a wide-legged position with your feet apart at a distance of one of your legs, with feet turned out at an angle.

2. Bend your knees to a 90-degree angle.

3. Reach your arms out to the sides and bend them up at a 90-degree angle, so your fingers are pointing up.

4. Keep your gaze looking forward.

5. Hold this pose for 8 to 10 full breaths.

6. To come out of this pose, bring your arms down, straighten your legs, and bring them back to the centerline of your body.

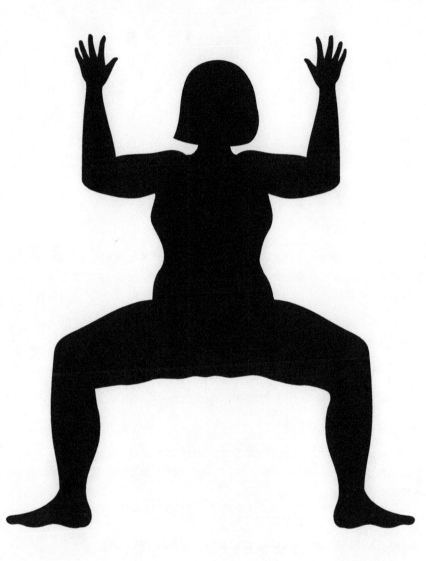

TIP: Add dynamic movement to this pose by straightening your legs, bringing your arms straight up, and gazing upward on your inhale, and then coming back down into the pose on the exhale. Repeat the cycle 15 to 25 times.

One-Legged Downward-Facing Dog: Adho Mukha Svanasana variation

BENEFITS: Strengthens the legs and pelvic floor muscles, improves balance

PRECAUTIONS: Use caution or avoid this pose if you have recently suffered an injury or have chronic pain in your legs, ankles, arms, or wrists.

INSTRUCTIONS:

1. Come onto your hands and knees into a tabletop position, keeping your hands and arms under your shoulders with palms flat on the ground and fingers spread apart, with your knees hip-width apart.

2. Tuck your toes, press into the ground with your hands and feet, and straighten your legs while lifting your hips up.

3. Press your heels down toward the ground; it is fine if they are slightly elevated.

4. Keep your legs straight and sit bones reaching upward.

5. Let your head relax and hang freely.

6. Lift your right leg up behind you, flexing the right foot and keeping the toes facing the floor. Keep the leg parallel to the ground or higher while keeping your hips even and square to the ground.

7. Hold this pose for 8 to 10 deep breaths.

8. Bring the foot back down into **Downward-Facing Dog** (page 56) and repeat with the other leg.

9. To come out of this pose, ensure both feet are back on the ground and gently come back into the tabletop position.

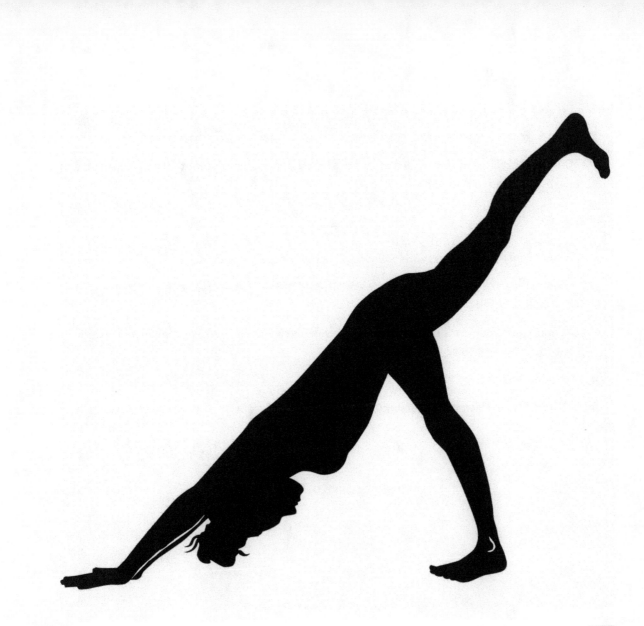

TIP: For extra resistance and strength training, add a resistance band to your ankles and alternate lifting your legs while wearing the band.

Fierce Pose: Utkatasana

BENEFITS: Builds strength in the legs, slightly releases the pelvic floor muscles

PRECAUTIONS: Use caution or avoid this pose if you have recently suffered an injury or have chronic pain in your legs or ankles.

INSTRUCTIONS:

1. Stand evenly on both feet, with your feet together and legs straight.

2. Bend both knees to about a 90-degree angle, and reach your arms above your head with your palms facing each other.

3. As you reach your arms up, sit your hips back as far as you can without falling backward, like you are about to sit on a chair.

4. Hold for 8 to 10 deep breaths.

5. To come out of this pose, straighten your legs and bring your arms down by your sides.

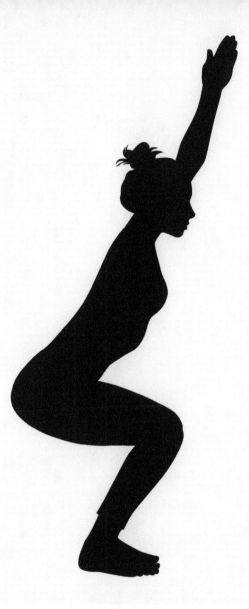

TIP: To add dynamic movement to this pose and to make it a bit easier to hold, straighten your legs on your inhale and then bend them on the exhale. Repeat the cycle 15 to 25 times.

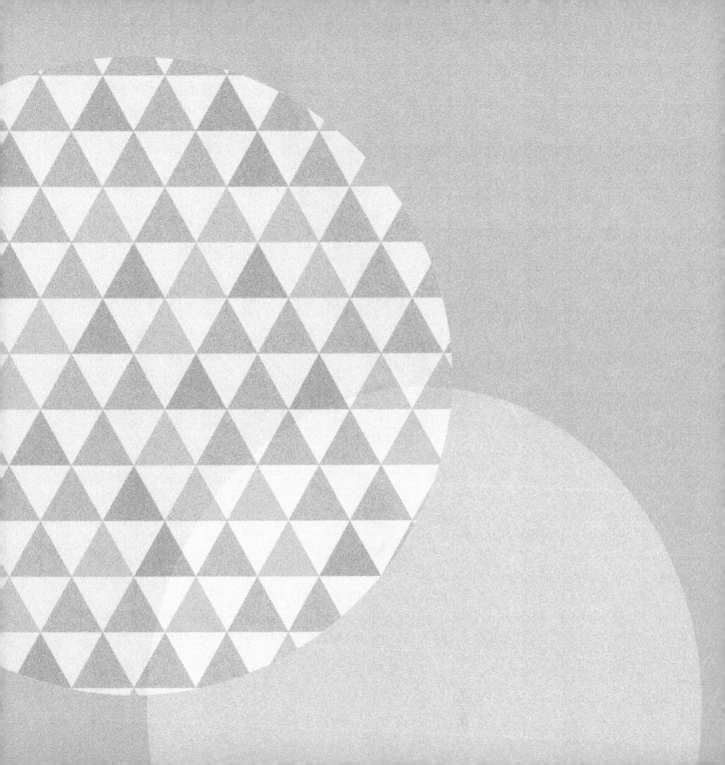

CHAPTER FIVE

Harmonizing Poses for the Pelvic Floor

In this chapter, I share yoga poses that relax and release the pelvic floor muscles to harmonize the connection between your body and the pelvic floor. These poses will stretch the muscles in your pelvic floor, while also helping you activate the parasympathetic nervous system, which aids in overall relaxation.

Reclined Easy Pose:
Supta Sukhasana

BENEFITS: Relaxes and releases the pelvic floor muscles

PRECAUTIONS: Use caution or avoid this pose if you have recently suffered an injury or have chronic pain in your legs, hips, knees, or back.

INSTRUCTIONS:

1. Sit on the ground with both sit bones evenly on the ground, and cross your right shin in front of your left, flexing both feet under your knees.

2. Engage your abdominal muscles and bring your hands to the ground behind you.

3. Gently and slowly lower your back to rest on the ground.

4. Reach your arms up toward your head, keeping them resting on the ground and your palms facing up toward the ceiling.

5. Hold for 15 to 30 full breaths.

6. To come out of this pose, uncross your legs, roll to the right side of your body, and use your hands to help yourself come up to a seated position.

7. Repeat this pose with the left shin crossed in front of the right if you would like to maintain symmetry in your body.

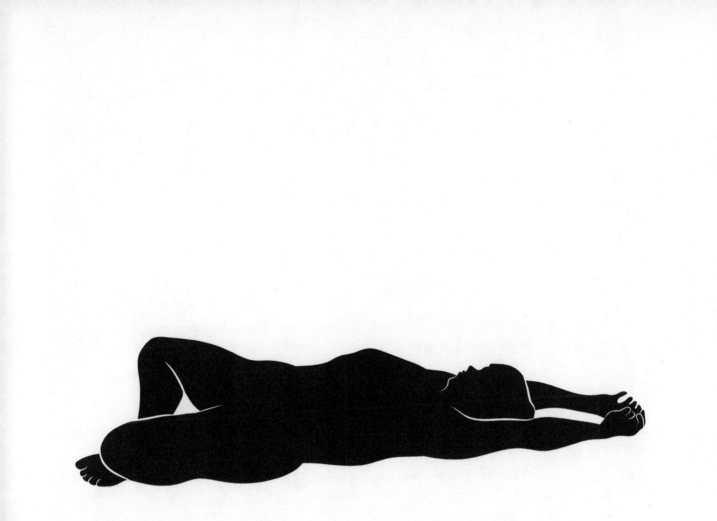

 TIP: Add a folded blanket or bolster under your back for support if resting all the way back on the ground is not possible for you at this time.

Reclined Bound Angle Pose: Supta Baddha Konasana

PROP: Bolster or folded blanket

BENEFITS: Relaxes and releases the pelvic floor muscles

PRECAUTIONS: Use caution or avoid this pose if you have recently suffered an injury or have chronic pain in your hips, legs, knees, or back.

INSTRUCTIONS:

1. Sit on the ground with both sit bones evenly on the ground, bending your legs and bringing your knees out to the sides and your feet to meet each other.

2. Bring your hands behind you, and gently lower your back onto a bolster or folded blanket so it supports your entire torso.

3. Place your hands down by your sides on the ground with palms facing up.

4. Hold for 15 to 30 deep breaths.

5. To come out of this pose, release your feet from each other and roll to the right, off the bolster or blanket.

6. Use your hands to help yourself come back up to a seated position.

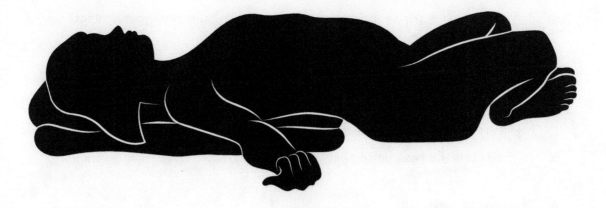

TIP: If your flexibility permits, try this pose without the bolster or blanket for an extra stretch.

Seated Twist:
Ardha Matsyendrasana

BENEFITS: Stretches the spine and lower back, helps relax the pelvic floor

PRECAUTIONS: Use caution or avoid this pose if you have recently suffered an injury or have chronic pain in your hips, legs, knees, or back.

INSTRUCTIONS:

1. Sit on the ground with both sit bones evenly on the ground. Bend your left leg, bringing the heel in toward your right sit bone.

2. Bend your right leg, point your knee up toward the ceiling, and cross your right foot over your left thigh.

3. On an inhale, twist your torso toward your right leg, and anchor your left elbow to the outer side of your right leg.

4. With your right hand on the ground behind you and your gaze over your right shoulder, hold this pose for 8 to 10 full breaths.

5. To come out of this pose, untwist your upper body and uncross your right leg from the left.

6. Repeat on the other side.

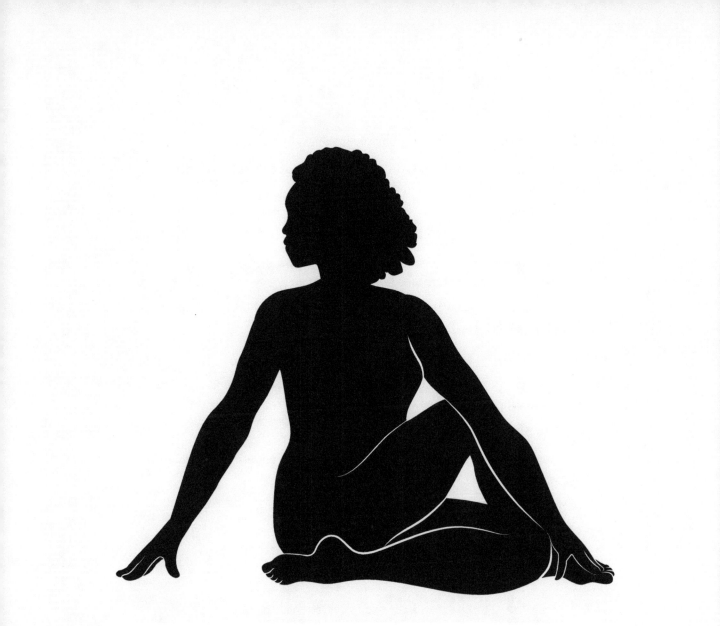

TIP: If you are not able to place your left elbow on the outer edge of your right thigh, hug the right leg with your left arm instead for a similar effect.

Marichi's Pose: Marichyasana 3

BENEFITS: Stretches the spine and lower back, helps relax the pelvic floor

PRECAUTIONS: Use caution or avoid this pose if you have recently suffered an injury or have chronic pain in your hips, legs, knees, or back.

INSTRUCTIONS:

1. Sit on the ground with both sit bones evenly on the ground, and stretch both legs out in front of you, with feet flexed and toes facing the ceiling.

2. Bend your right leg and place the bottom of your right foot on the ground next to your left leg with your right knee up toward the ceiling.

3. Inhale and twist the upper body toward the right leg.

4. Wrap your left arm around the right leg and bring the right arm around you until your hands meet at your back, clasped together.

5. Hold for 8 to 10 full breaths.

6. To come out of this pose, unclasp your hands and release your arms. Straighten your right leg and untwist your torso.

7. Repeat on the other side.

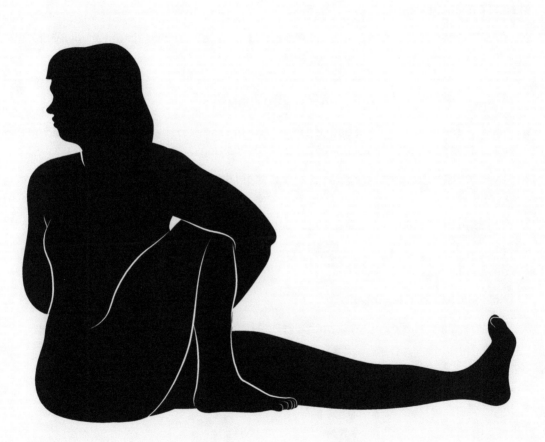

TIP: If your flexibility currently does not permit you to wrap your arms around your bent leg, do the same arm position as for **Seated Twist** (page 86).

Reclined Twist:
Supta Matsyendrasana variation

BENEFITS: Initiates the relaxation response, stretches the lower back

PRECAUTIONS: Use caution or avoid this pose if you have recently suffered an injury or have chronic pain in your hips, legs, knees, or back.

INSTRUCTIONS:

1. Lie flat on the ground, bend both legs, and hug the knees in toward the chest. Hold on to your shins with both hands or hold on to the hamstrings.

2. Take both bent legs and bring them over to the right side of your body and rest them on the ground.

3. Reach your arms out to the sides and keep your palms flat on the ground.

4. Twist your upper body and bring your gaze over to the left as you rest your head on the ground.

5. Hold for 15 to 25 deep breaths.

6. To come out of this pose, bring both legs and head back to center and repeat on the other side.

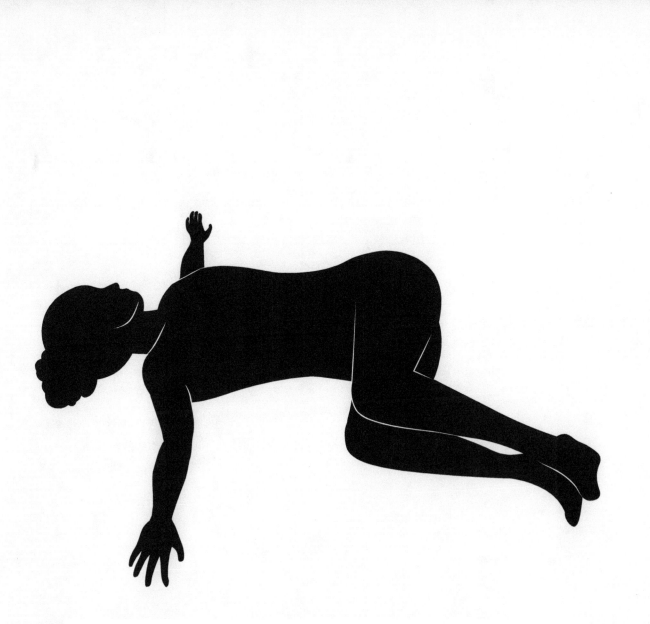

TIP: For a deeper thigh stretch for the leg on top, straighten that leg in its place and hold on to it with the opposite hand to hold the stretch.

Reclined Single Leg Stretch: Supta Padangusthasana

BENEFITS: Stretches the legs and pelvic floor muscles, increasing flexibility

PRECAUTIONS: Use caution or avoid this pose if you have recently suffered an injury or have chronic pain in your hips, legs, knees, or back.

INSTRUCTIONS:

1. Lie flat on the ground with your legs straight and feet flexed.

2. Raise your right leg, bending it in toward your chest while you hold on to your shin. Keep the left leg on the ground.

3. Straighten your right leg and hold on to the foot or calf muscle with both hands. You should feel a stretch in the back of your right leg and slightly in the front of your left leg.

4. Hold for 8 to 10 deep breaths.

5. To come out of this pose, release your right leg and bring it back down to the ground.

6. Repeat on the other side.

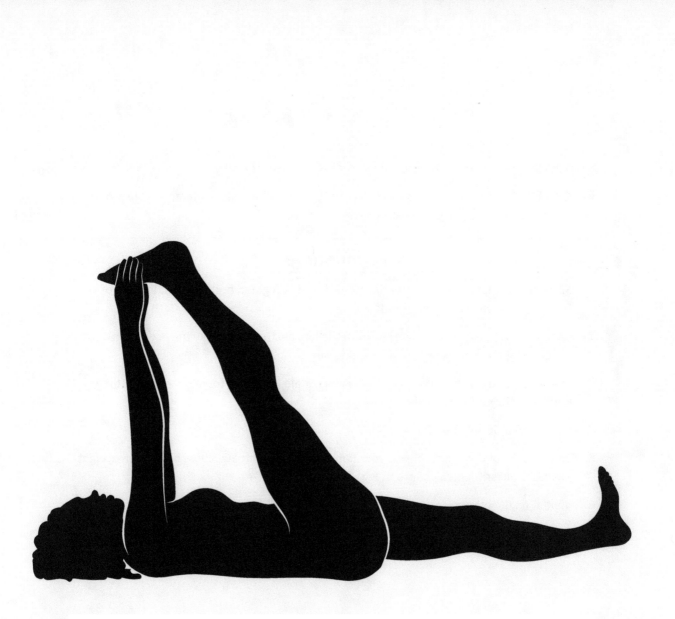

 TIP: If you have trouble reaching your foot, use a yoga strap by placing it around your foot on your raised leg and hold on to the strap instead.

Head to Knee Forward Bend: Janu Sirsasana

BENEFITS: Stretches the legs, hips, and lower back, relaxes the pelvic floor muscles

PRECAUTIONS: Use caution or avoid this pose if you have recently suffered an injury or have chronic pain in your hips, legs, knees, or back.

INSTRUCTIONS:

1. Sit with both sit bones evenly on the ground, and straighten both legs out in front of you. Flex your feet and keep your toes facing up.

2. Bend your right leg, turn the leg out from the hip, and rest the pinky toe-side of your right leg on the ground, so your knee is pointing out.

3. Inhale to lengthen your spine, and while you exhale, fold your torso over your left leg, holding on to your foot, ankle, or shin with both hands.

4. Hold for 8 to 10 full breaths.

5. To come out of this pose, release your hands from your left leg, come back to an upright position, and straighten your right leg.

6. Repeat on the other side.

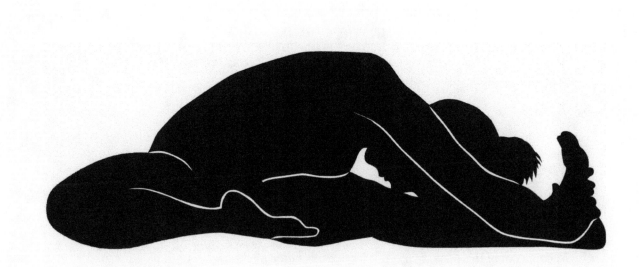

TIP: If you experience knee pain, place the bottom of your bent leg on the shin of the straightened leg. Do not place your foot on your knee joint.

Revolved Head to Knee Pose:
Janu Sirsasana variation

BENEFITS: Stretches the legs, hips, and lower back, relaxes the pelvic floor muscles

PRECAUTIONS: Use caution or avoid this pose if you have recently suffered an injury or have chronic pain in your hips, legs, knees, or back.

INSTRUCTIONS:

1. Sit with both sit bones evenly on the ground, and stretch your left leg out to the side with your knee and toes facing up.

2. Bend your right leg to bring the heel in toward the pelvis.

3. Inhale to lengthen your spine, and exhale to fold your torso over toward the left leg, keeping your shoulders facing forward.

4. You can reach the right arm up on a diagonal or touch your left toes if your flexibility permits you to do so.

5. Hold for 8 to 10 deep breaths.

6. To come out of this pose, bring your hand back, come back to an upright position, and repeat on the other side.

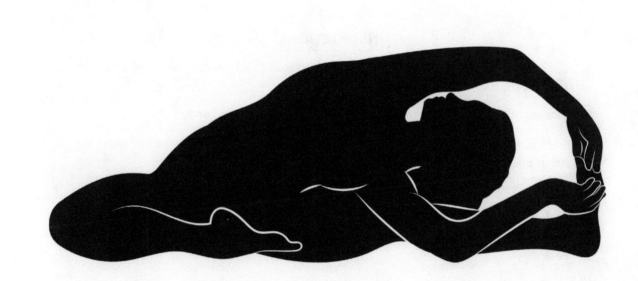

TIP: Use a yoga strap to hold on to the foot of your straightened leg if you are unable to reach your foot with your hand at this time.

Reclined Straddle: Supta Samakonasana

BENEFITS: Stretches the inner thighs and pelvic floor muscles

PRECAUTIONS: Use caution or avoid this pose if you have recently suffered an injury or have chronic pain in your hips, legs, knees, or back.

INSTRUCTIONS:

1. Lying flat on the ground, hug both legs in toward your chest, holding on to the shins with both hands.

2. Straighten your legs out to the sides, holding your toes in your hands.

3. Keep your lower back on the ground, resisting the urge to round the spine and curve the pelvis under.

4. Hold for 8 to 10 deep breaths.

5. To come out of this pose, gently release your hands from your feet and bring your legs back in toward your chest. Release your hands from your legs and bring your legs back down.

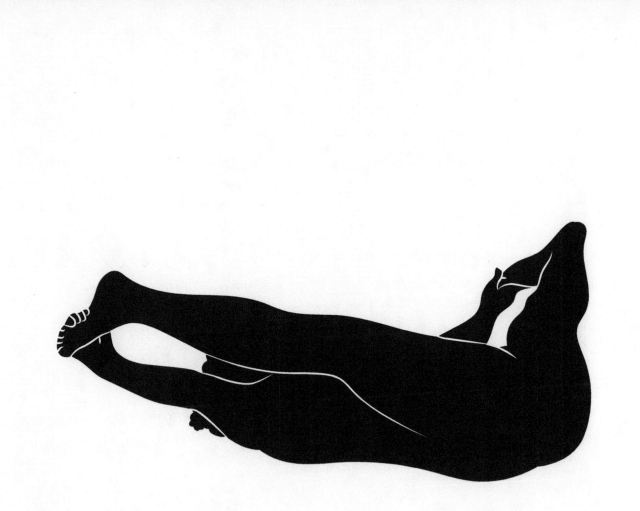

TIP: Do this pose with your legs resting against a wall for more support if that feels more comfortable for you.

Knees to Chest Pose: Apanasana

BENEFITS: Stretches the hamstrings and gluteus muscles, which support the pelvic floor

PRECAUTIONS: Use caution or avoid this pose if you have recently suffered an injury or have chronic pain in your hips, legs, knees, or back.

INSTRUCTIONS:

1. Lie flat on your back and bend your legs, flexing your feet.

2. Hug your knees in toward your chest, holding them with your arms in a hugging position or holding on to your shins with both hands.

3. Hold for 15 to 25 deep breaths.

4. To come out of this pose, release your hands from your legs and bring your legs back down.

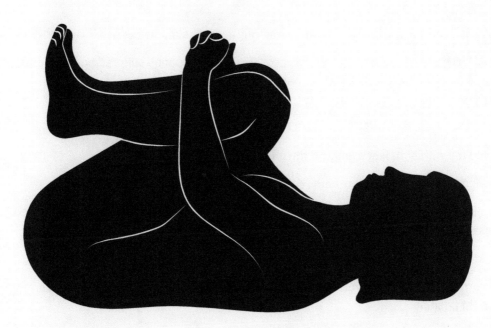

  TIP: Hold on to your hamstrings with your hands instead of holding your shins if that is more comfortable for you.

Straight-Legged Standing Forward Fold: Uttanasana

BENEFITS: Stretches the lower back and hamstrings, which support the pelvic floor

PRECAUTIONS: Use caution or avoid this pose if you have recently suffered an injury or have chronic pain in your hips, legs, knees, or back.

INSTRUCTIONS:

1. Stand tall with both feet evenly on the ground.

2. Straighten both legs and flex both feet, keeping your toes facing the ceiling.

3. Inhale to lengthen the spine, and while exhaling, fold your torso over your straightened legs, holding on to the feet, ankles, or shins.

4. Hold for 8 to 10 deep breaths.

5. To come out of this pose, release your hands from your legs and come back to an upright position.

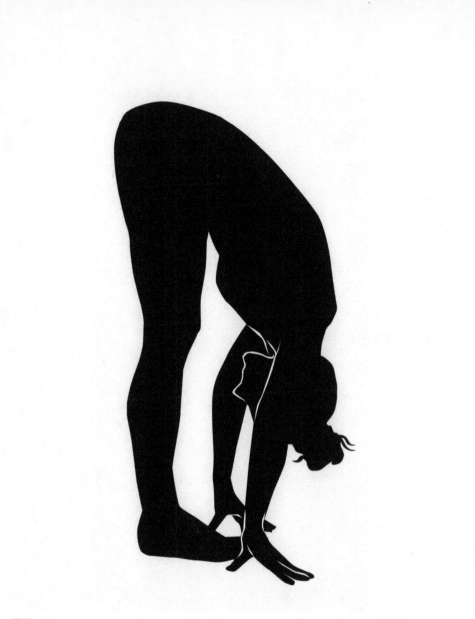

 TIP: Use a yoga strap by wrapping the strap around your feet and holding on to the strap ends with both hands if that is more comfortable for you.

Reclined Cow Face Pose: Supta Gomukhasana

BENEFITS: Stretches the outer thighs, relaxes the pelvic floor muscles

PRECAUTIONS: Use caution or avoid this pose if you have recently suffered an injury or have chronic pain in your hips, legs, knees, or back.

INSTRUCTIONS:

1. Lying flat on the ground, hug both legs in toward your chest.

2. Cross your right thigh over your left thigh and hold on to your ankles with your hands, keeping your legs up and in toward your chest.

3. Hold for 8 to 10 deep breaths.

4. To come out of this pose, release your hands from your ankles and uncross your legs.

5. Repeat, crossing your legs on the other side.

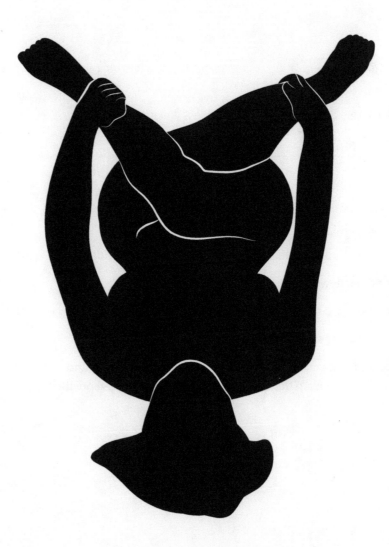

TIP: If you have knee pain in this pose, modify it by doing the **Knees to Chest Pose** (page 100) instead and holding on to your hamstrings with both hands.

Legs Up the Wall: Viparita Karani

BENEFITS: Initiates the relaxation response in the body, allowing the pelvic floor to release and relax

PRECAUTIONS: Use caution or avoid this pose if you have recently suffered an injury or have chronic pain in your hips, legs, knees, or back.

INSTRUCTIONS:

1. Lie flat on the ground with your sit bones up against the edge of a wall. Fold a blanket and place it under your lower back for support and proper alignment.

2. Stretch your legs up the wall and keep them relaxed, hip-width apart.

3. Place your arms down by your sides with palms facing up.

4. Close your eyes and breathe in and out through your nose, focusing on your breath.

5. Hold for 25 to 45 deep, full breaths.

6. To come out of this pose, bend your legs, roll to the right side, and use your hands to help yourself come away from the wall and into an upright seated position.

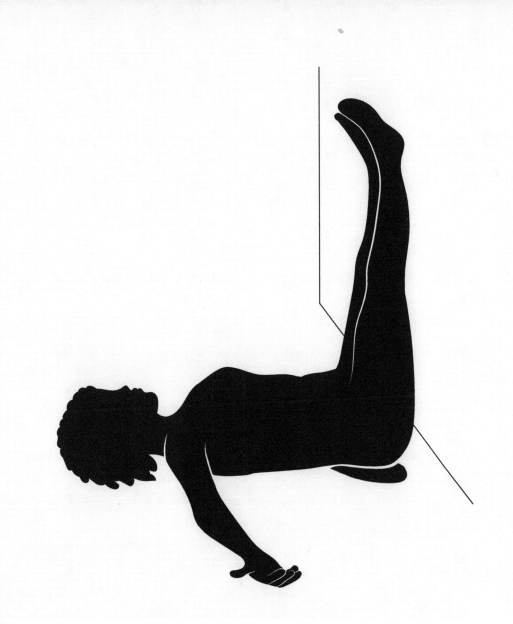

TIP: To keep your legs from splaying outward while you relax in this pose, use a yoga strap set at your shins to keep the legs hip-width apart.

Corpse Pose: Savasana

BENEFITS: Initiates the relaxation response in the body, providing the pelvic floor with deep relaxation

PRECAUTIONS: Use caution or avoid this pose if you have recently suffered an injury or have chronic pain in your hips, legs, knees, or back.

INSTRUCTIONS:

1. Lie flat with your back on the ground, your body completely relaxed, and your palms facing up.

2. Keep your legs apart from each other and relax them completely.

3. Close your eyes and breathe in and out through your nose, focusing on your breath.

4. Hold for 25 to 45 deep, full breaths.

5. To come out of this pose, gently bring motion back into your body by wiggling your hands and feet.

6. Roll to the right side with your knees bent and your arm under your head for support. Remain there for a few deep breaths.

7. Use your hands on the ground to help yourself come into an upright seated position.

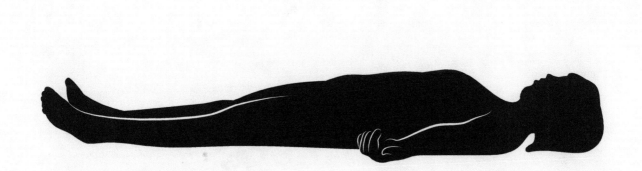

 TIP: If you have lower back pain in this pose, place a rolled blanket under your knees to alleviate the pressure.

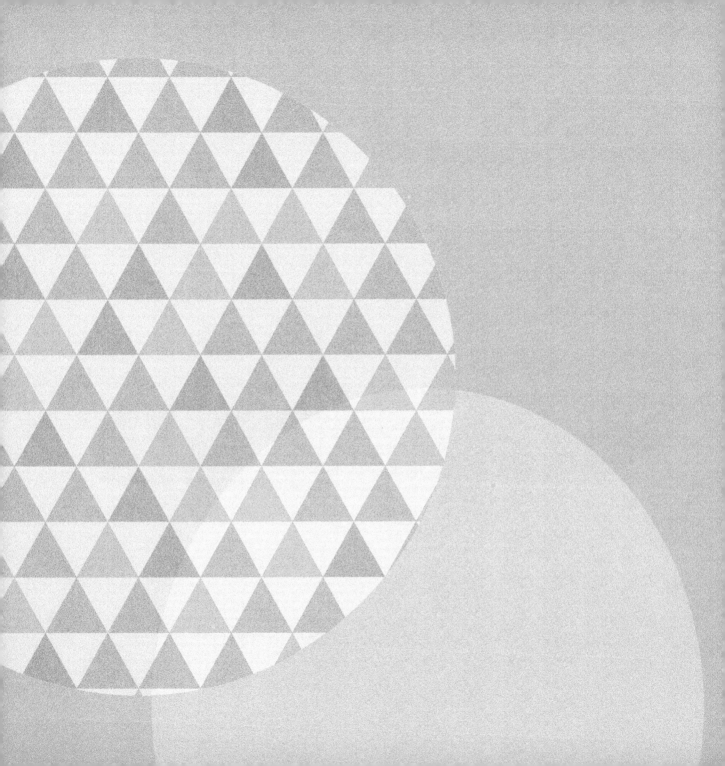

CHAPTER SIX

Sequences to Support the Pelvic Floor

In this chapter, you'll find 10 yoga sequences utilizing the yoga poses from previous chapters that you can practice at home. These yoga sequences will help you energize, stretch, release, heal, ground, and reconnect to your pelvic floor. Regularly practicing these yoga routines will also help improve your sexual health, self-esteem, and overall well-being.

Energizing the Pelvic Floor

This sequence can help energize the pelvic floor and your overall body. With regular practice, this sequence will help you feel stronger, more self-confident, and empowered. Practice this if you are feeling weak in the pelvic floor area and looking for more strength and energy.

INSTRUCTIONS:

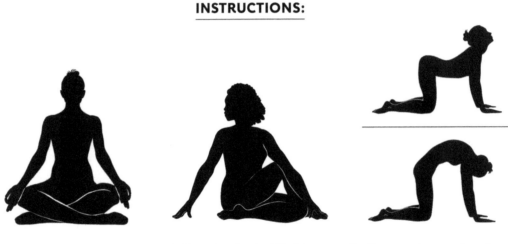

1. Begin in **Easy Pose** (page 32).

2. Practice **Seated Twist** (page 86) on the right side, followed by the left.

3. Come onto your hands and knees and move through **Cat/Cow** (page 40).

 TIP: Don't be afraid to use yoga props or prop substitutions during your practice. They are a great tool to help you feel more comfortable in the poses and achieve the goal of the pose in a safe way.

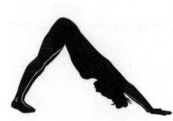 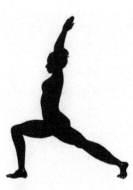 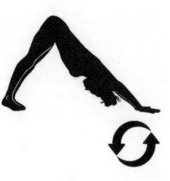

4. Bring your spine back to neutral and move the hips up for **Downward-Facing Dog** (page 56).

5. Step your right leg forward between your hands for **High Lunge** (page 46).

6. Ground your hands and step the right foot back for **Downward-Facing Dog**.

7. Repeat steps 5 and 6 on the other side.

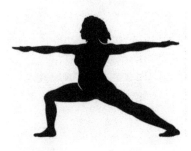 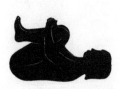 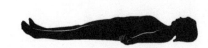

8. Step the right foot up and come into **Warrior 2** (page 58). Repeat on the other side.

9. Lie back flat on the ground and fold into **Knees to Chest Pose** (page 100).

10. Release the legs and relax into **Corpse Pose** (page 108).

Stretching the Pelvic Floor

This sequence is designed to stretch, lengthen, and release the muscles in your pelvic floor. If you're feeling tight in that area and in need of some comfort by releasing the muscles, this is a great sequence.

INSTRUCTIONS:

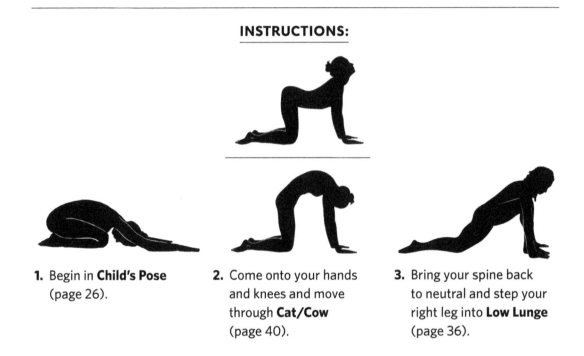

1. Begin in **Child's Pose** (page 26).

2. Come onto your hands and knees and move through **Cat/Cow** (page 40).

3. Bring your spine back to neutral and step your right leg into **Low Lunge** (page 36).

 TIP: In **Reclined Pigeon Pose**, it's okay for the shin to be diagonal instead of horizontal, with your heel slightly inward toward your pelvis.

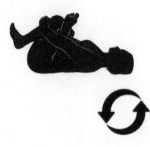

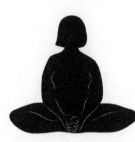

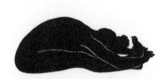

4. Transition into **Reclined Pigeon Pose** (page 44) on the right side.

5. Repeat steps 3 and 4 on the other side.

6. Release the legs and sit into **Bound Angle Pose** (page 34).

7. Release the legs into **Straight-Legged Seated Forward Fold** (page 50).

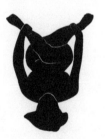

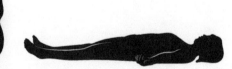

8. Move into **Reclined Cow Face Pose** (page 104) on the right side, followed by the left.

9. Stretch out the arms and legs into **Reclined Straddle** (page 98).

10. Release the legs and relax into **Corpse Pose** (page 108).

Strengthening the Pelvic Floor

This sequence can help you strengthen your pelvic floor muscles. If you have been told or you feel that your pelvic floor muscles are weak, this is a great sequence to tighten and build muscle strength in that area.

INSTRUCTIONS:

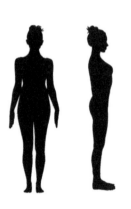 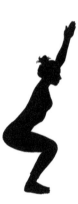 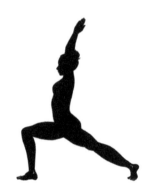

1. Come to standing evenly on both feet in **Mountain Pose** (page 54).

2. Sit your hips into **Fierce Pose** (page 78).

3. Keeping your core and legs engaged, step your left leg backward, coming into **High Lunge** (page 46) on the right side.

TIP: Legs Up the Wall (page 106) and **Corpse Pose** (page 108) can be added to any of the sequences including this one. Feel free to do either one, depending on which you prefer or feel like doing in the moment. Both poses activate the same relaxation response in your body.

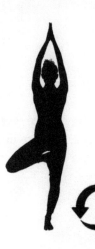

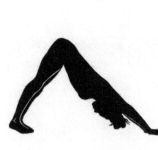

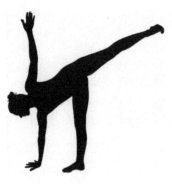

4. Bring your left leg forward to meet the right foot and move into **Tree Pose** (page 66) on the right side.

5. Repeat steps 3 and 4 on the other side.

6. Plant both feet firmly on the ground and transition into **Downward-Facing Dog** (page 56).

7. Stand up and spread the legs to come into **Half-Moon Pose** (page 64) on the right side, followed by the left.

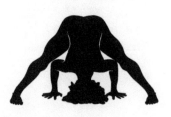

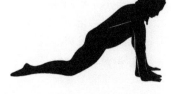

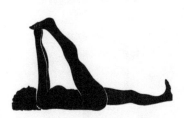

8. Come into **Standing Wide-Legged Forward Fold** (page 48).

9. Come down onto the ground for **Low Lunge** (page 36) on the right side, followed by the left.

10. Lie flat on the ground and move into **Reclined Single Leg Stretch** (page 92) on the right side, followed by the left.

Relaxing the Pelvic Floor

This sequence can help you relax your pelvic floor muscles. It's a restorative yoga routine that will help you simultaneously focus your mind and relax your muscles. Practice this if you need to wind down and bring some relaxation into your life. Prepare a bolster or stacked blankets and have them nearby.

INSTRUCTIONS:

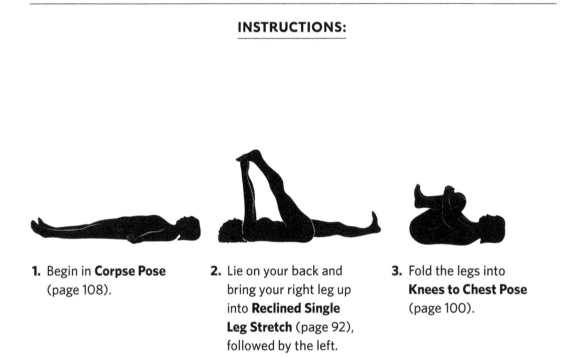

1. Begin in **Corpse Pose** (page 108).

2. Lie on your back and bring your right leg up into **Reclined Single Leg Stretch** (page 92), followed by the left.

3. Fold the legs into **Knees to Chest Pose** (page 100).

TIP: You can relax more by spending a bit more time in each pose, closing your eyes, and focusing more on your breath. Also, if there is a certain pose in this sequence that does not feel good in your body, modify it or skip it. You can always come back to it another time when you feel more ready for it.

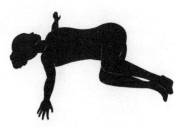

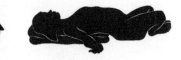

4. Bring the knees down into **Reclined Twist** (page 90) on the right side.

5. Come back to center and into **Reclined Pigeon Pose** (page 44) on the right side.

6. Repeat steps 4 and 5 on the other side.

7. Lower the legs into **Reclined Bound Angle Pose** (page 84).

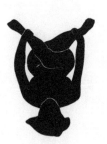

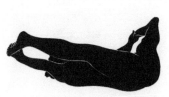

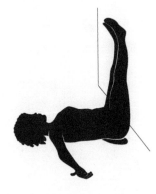

8. Bring the legs up into **Reclined Cow Face Pose** (page 104) on the right side, followed by the left.

9. Stretch out the legs and arms into **Reclined Straddle** (page 98).

10. Release the legs, find a wall, and relax into **Legs Up the Wall** (page 106).

Tightening the Pelvic Floor

This yoga sequence is designed to tighten your pelvic floor muscles. If you feel that you need to tighten things back up after childbirth or if you just have naturally loose and weak pelvic floor muscles, this is a great sequence to practice to gain more control of the area.

INSTRUCTIONS:

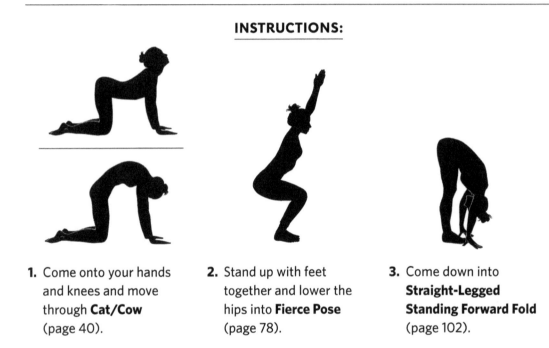

1. Come onto your hands and knees and move through **Cat/Cow** (page 40).

2. Stand up with feet together and lower the hips into **Fierce Pose** (page 78).

3. Come down into **Straight-Legged Standing Forward Fold** (page 102).

TIP: Since this sequence is quite intense, you can add another restorative pose at the end, such as **Corpse Pose** (page 108).

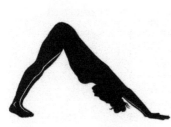

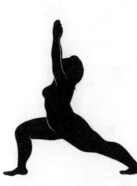

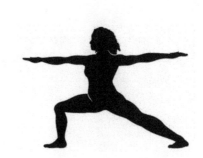

4. Place your hands evenly on the ground and step the feet back for **Downward-Facing Dog** (page 56).

5. Step the right foot up and come into **Warrior 1** (page 70) on the right.

6. Lower the arms into **Warrior 2** (page 58) on the right.

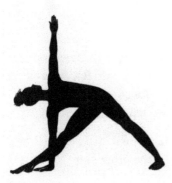

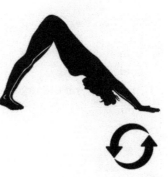

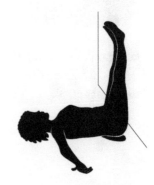

7. Straighten the right leg for **Triangle Pose** (page 60) on the right.

8. Come into table-top position for **Downward-Facing Dog.**

9. Repeat steps 5 to 8 on the other side.

10. Release from pose, find a wall, and relax into **Legs Up the Wall** (page 106).

Releasing the Pelvic Floor

If you are holding a lot of tension in your pelvic floor muscles and need some release to relieve that tension, try this sequence to release that tight pelvic floor.

INSTRUCTIONS:

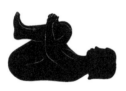 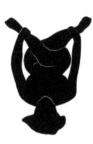 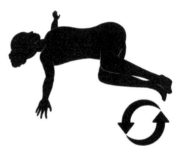

1. Lie flat on the ground and fold into **Knees to Chest Pose** (page 100).

2. Transition into **Reclined Cow Face Pose** (page 104) on the right.

3. Uncross the legs and come into **Reclined Twist** (page 90) on the right side.

4. Repeat steps 2 and 3 on the other side.

 TIP: If you have extra time, add this sequence to the end of a strengthening sequence for a more well-rounded and balanced practice.

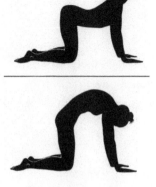

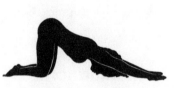

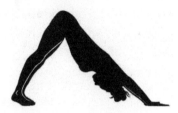

5. Come up onto your hands and knees and move through **Cat/Cow** (page 40).

6. Go from tabletop position into **Melting Heart** (page 42).

7. Spread your fingers apart and come into **Downward-Facing Dog** (page 56).

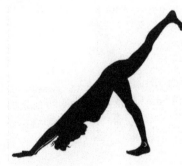

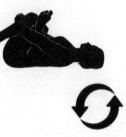

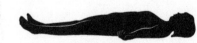

8. Lift your right leg into **One-Legged Downward-Facing Dog** (page 76).

9. Lie on your back and move into **Reclined Pigeon Pose** (page 44) on the right.

10. Repeat steps 7 and 9 on the other side.

11. Release the legs and relax into **Corpse Pose** (page 108).

Reconnecting to Your Pelvic Floor

This yoga sequence can help you reconnect to your pelvic floor. It will help invigorate the muscles in that area and allow you to feel their presence more in your body. Practice this routine regularly to gain more of a sense of your pelvic floor and deepen your connection to that area of your body.

INSTRUCTIONS:

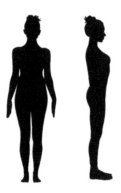

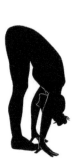

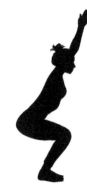

1. Come to standing evenly on both feet in **Mountain Pose** (page 54).

2. Come into **Straight-Legged Standing Forward Fold** (page 102).

3. Straighten up, bring your feet together and move into **Fierce Pose** (page 78).

TIP: Swap **Seated Twist** (page 86) for **Marichi's Pose** if you would like a deeper thigh stretch. Use your best judgment while practicing yoga and do what works best for you.

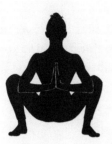

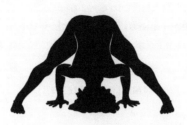

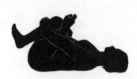

4. Spread your legs mat-width apart and come into **Wide-Legged Squat** (page 30).

5. Spread your legs farther out into **Standing Wide-Legged Forward Fold** (page 48).

6. Lie on your back and come into **Reclined Pigeon Pose** (page 44) on the right side, followed by the left.

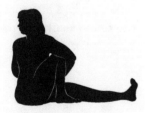

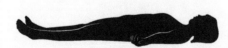

7. Sit on the ground and move into **Marichi's Pose** (page 88) on the right side, followed by the left.

8. Lie flat and relax into **Corpse Pose** (page 108).

This yoga sequence is designed to help you ease pelvic floor tension and pressure. If you feel a lot of pressure in the pelvic area due to tight muscles, this is a great routine to add to your yoga practice regularly. Prepare a bolster or stacked blankets and have them nearby.

INSTRUCTIONS:

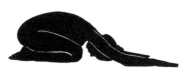 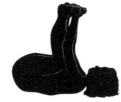 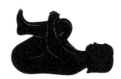

1. Come into tabletop position and move into **Child's Pose** (page 26).

2. Lie on your back and come into **Happy Baby** (page 28).

3. Bend your legs and come into **Knees to Chest Pose** (page 100).

TIP: If you do not have a clear wall space to practice this sequence, replace **Legs Up the Wall** with **Corpse Pose** (page 108). It achieves a similar feeling within the body and allows you to relax without needing a wall.

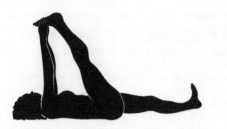

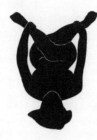

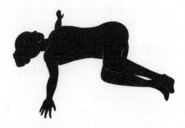

4. Flex your feet and move into **Reclined Single Leg Stretch** (page 92) on the right side, followed by the left.

5. Hug both legs in and do **Reclined Cow Face Pose** (page 104) on the right side, followed by the left.

6. Hug both legs in and do **Reclined Twist** (page 90) on the right side, followed by the left.

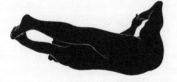

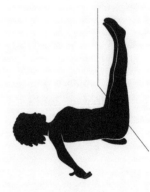

7. Hold the shins and move into **Reclined Straddle** (page 98).

8. Sit on the ground and come into **Reclined Bound Angle Pose** (page 84).

9. Release the legs, find a wall, and relax into **Legs Up the Wall** (page 106).

Feeling Grounded in Your Pelvic Floor

This sequence can help you feel more grounded in your pelvic floor area. At times we can feel like we have lost control in certain areas of our body, including our pelvic floor. If you feel this way, this sequence may be able to help you calm down and feel more stable in that area.

INSTRUCTIONS:

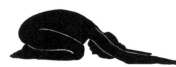
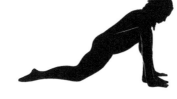
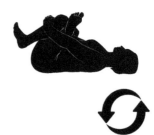

1. Begin in tabletop position and move into **Child's Pose** (page 26).

2. Come into tabletop position and move into **Low Lunge** on the right side (page 36).

3. Lie back into **Reclined Pigeon Pose** on the right side (page 44).

4. Repeat steps 2 and 3 on the other side.

TIP: Substitute **Goddess Pose** (page 74) for the **Wide-Legged Squat** if you experience knee pain in any way. They are both squatting wide-legged poses, but Goddess Pose will put less pressure on your knees.

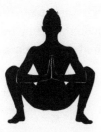

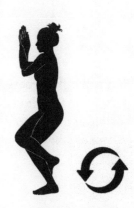

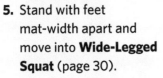

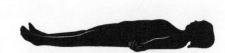

5. Stand with feet mat-width apart and move into **Wide-Legged Squat** (page 30).

6. Bring your feet together into **Tree Pose** on the right side (page 66).

7. Stand tall and transition into **Eagle Pose** (page 68) on the right side.

8. Repeat steps 6 and 7 on the other side.

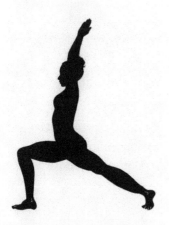

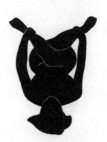

9. Move into tabletop position and do **High Lunge** (page 46) on the right side, followed by the left.

10. Lie on your back and move into **Reclined Cow Face Pose** (page 104) on the right side, followed by the left.

11. Release the legs and relax into **Corpse Pose** (page 108).

Pelvic Floor Yoga for Pregnancy

This pelvic floor routine is great to practice if you are pregnant and looking to prepare your pelvic floor for labor. This gentle routine will help you release any tension you may be holding in the pelvic area while also adding some relaxation into your entire body. Prepare a bolster or stacked blankets and have them nearby.

INSTRUCTIONS:

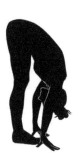

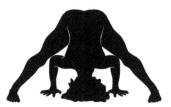

1. Come to standing evenly on both feet in **Mountain Pose** (page 54).

2. Stand tall and move into **Straight-Legged Standing Forward Fold** (page 102).

3. Slowly spread your legs apart into **Standing Wide-Legged Forward Fold** (page 48).

TIP: If you are pregnant, practice this and any other sequence or pose with caution. Simply because someone says it is "safe for pregnancy" does not necessarily mean it is right for you in the moment. If anything makes you feel uncomfortable, in pain, or just not right, listen to your body and stop what you are doing.

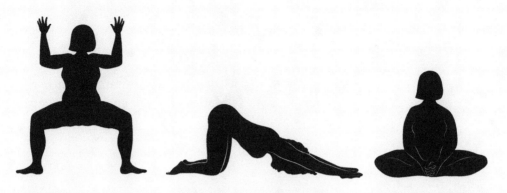

4. Keep legs wide for **Goddess Pose** (page 74).

5. Come into tabletop position to do **Melting Heart** (page 42).

6. Sit on the ground in **Bound Angle Pose** (page 34).

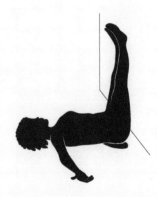

7. Lie back into **Reclined Easy Pose** (page 82) with the support of a bolster or stacked blankets.

8. Sit on the ground and transition into **Reclined Bound Angle Pose** (page 84).

9. Release the legs, find a wall, and relax into **Legs Up the Wall** (page 106).

Resources

Books

Chair Yoga: Accessible Sequences to Build Strength, Flexibility, and Inner Calm by Christina D'Arrigo

Essential Chakra Yoga: Poses to Balance, Heal, and Energize the Body and Mind by Christina D'Arrigo

Evidence-Based Physical Therapy for the Pelvic Floor: Bridging Science and Clinical Practice by Kari Bo, PT, PhD, Bary Berghmans, PhD, MSc, RPt, Siv Morkved, PT, MSc, PhD, and Marijke Van Kampen, PhD

Restorative Yoga for Beginners: Gentle Poses for Relaxation and Healing by Julia Clarke

Restoring the Pelvic Floor: How Kegel Exercises, Vaginal Training, and Relaxation Solve Incontinence, Constipation, and Heal Pelvic Pain to Avoid Surgery by Amanda A. Olson

Online

American Physical Therapy Association: APTA.org

International Pelvic Pain Society: PelvicPain.org

International Society for the Study of Women's Health: ISSWSH.org

National Vulvodynia Association: NVA.org

Author Links

Facebook: Facebook.com/chriskayoga

Instagram: @chriskayoga

Membership site: ChriskaYoga.vhx.tv

Website: ChriskaYoga.com

YouTube: YouTube.com/user/chriskayoga

References

Bryant, Kelly. "The Fascinating History of the Kegel." *Kelly Bryant Wellness*. Accessed September 4, 2021. KellyBryantWellness.com/2020/03/01/history-of-the-kegel.

D'Arrigo, Christina. *Essential Chakra Yoga: Poses to Balance, Heal, and Energize the Body and Mind*. Emeryville, CA: Rockridge Press, 2020.

Kaminoff, Leslie, and Amy Matthews. *Yoga Anatomy*. Champaign, IL: Human Kinetics, 2021.

Physiopedia. "The Pelvic Floor—Overview and Function." Accessed September 4, 2021. Physio-pedia.com/Pelvic_Floor_Anatomy.

YogaJournal.com.

Index

Acknowledgments

Thank you, once again, to Callisto Media for providing me with the opportunity to share my knowledge of yoga with more people. Thank you to Eun H. Jeong for your help and guidance throughout this process.

Thank you to my parents, Lisa and Joe, for babysitting and for your lifetime of support. Thank you to my husband, Barry, for all of your love and support throughout this process and beyond.

Thank you so much to the members of my Yoga With Christina online community for your kindness and support over the past seven years.

Last, but not least, thank you to my daughter, Lucy. My pelvic floor will never be the same, but I wouldn't have it any other way. I'm so proud and honored to be your mom.

About the Author

 Christina D'Arrigo is a 500 hour–trained yoga teacher and former dancer/choreographer from New York City. As a former attendee of LaGuardia High School of Music & Art and Performing Arts in New York City, D'Arrigo received her specialized high school diploma in dance. She then went on to study dance further in Los Angeles and London, where she received her bachelor's and master's degrees in dance and choreography. Upon her return to New York City, D'Arrigo completed her 500-hour yoga teacher training and began teaching yoga classes live and online for thousands of people all over the world via the YouTube channel *Yoga With Christina—ChriskaYoga* and various other platforms.

Printed in the USA
CPSIA information can be obtained
at www.ICGtesting.com
CBHW052003010424
6165CB00004B/7